INTERVENTIONAL CARDIOLOGY CLINICS

www.interventional.theclinics.com

Editor-in-Chief

MATTHEW J. PRICE

Hot Topics in Interventional Cardiology

October 2019 • Volume 8 • Number 4

ELSEVIER

1600 John F. Kennedy Boulevard • Suite 1800 • Philadelphia, Pennsylvania, 19103-2899

http://www.theclinics.com

INTERVENTIONAL CARDIOLOGY CLINICS Volume 8, Number 4
October 2019 ISSN 2211-7458, ISBN-13: 978-0-323-71229-3

Editor: Lauren Boyle
Developmental Editor: Donald Mumford

Interventional Cardiology Clinics (ISSN 2211-7458) is published quarterly by Elsevier Inc., 360 Park Avenue South, New York, NY 10010-1710. Months of issue are January, April, July, and October. Subscription prices are USD 203 per year for US individuals, USD 474 for US institutions, USD 100 per year for US students, USD 204 per year for Canadian individuals, USD 565 for Canadian institutions, USD 150 per year for Canadian students, USD 296 per year for international individuals, USD 565 for international institutions, and USD 150 per year for international students. To receive student/resident rate, orders must be accompanied by name of affiliated institution, date of term, and the *signature* of program/residency coordinator on institution letterhead. Orders will be billed at individual rate until proof of status is received. Foreign air speed delivery is included in all *Clinics* subscription prices. All prices are subject to change without notice. **POSTMASTER:** Send address changes to *Interventional Cardiology Clinics*, Elsevier Health Sciences Division, Subscription Customer Service, 3251 Riverport Lane, Maryland Heights, MO 63043. **Customer Service: Telephone: 1-800-654-2452** (U.S. and Canada); **1-314-447-8871** (outside U.S. and Canada). **Fax: 1-314-447-8029. E-mail: journalscustomerservice-usa@elsevier.com (for print support); journalsonlinesupport-usa@elsevier.com (for online support).**

Reprints. For copies of 100 or more of articles in this publication, please contact the Commercial Reprints Department, Elsevier Inc., 360 Park Avenue South, New York, NY 10010-1710. Tel.: 212-633-3874; Fax: 212-633-3820; E-mail: reprints@elsevier.com.

CONTRIBUTORS

EDITOR-IN-CHIEF

MATTHEW J. PRICE, MD
Director, Cardiac Catheterization Laboratory,
Division of Cardiovascular Diseases, Scripps
Clinic, La Jolla, California, USA

AUTHORS

HARSH AGRAWAL, MD, FACP, FACC,
RPVI, FSCAI
Clinical Instructor, Division of Cardiology,
University of California, San Francisco, San
Francisco, California, USA

DOMINICK J. ANGIOLILLO, MD, PhD
Division of Cardiology, University of Florida
College of Medicine, Jacksonville, Florida,
USA

ANGELOS ARFARAS-MELAINIS, MD
Clinical Research Fellow, Second Cardiology
Department, National and Kapodistrian
University of Athens, Attikon University
Hospital, Athens, Greece

PIERA CAPRANZANO, MD, PhD
Division of Cardiology, CAST Policlinico
Hospital, University of Catania, Catania,
Italy

GEORGE D. DANGAS, MD, PhD
The Zena and Michael A. Wiener
Cardiovascular Institute, Professor of
Medicine, Icahn School of Medicine at Mount
Sinai, Director of Cardiovascular Innovation,
Mount Sinai Medical Center, New York, New
York, USA

MARVIN H. ENG, MD
Center for Structural Heart Disease, Structural
Heart Disease Fellowship Director, Director of
Research for the Center for Structural Heart
Disease, Henry Ford Hospital, Detroit,
Michigan, USA

BRUNO FRANCAVIGLIA, MD
Division of Cardiology, CAST Policlinico
Hospital, University of Catania, Catania,
Italy

TIBERIO M. FRISOLI, MD
Henry Ford Hospital, Detroit, Michigan, USA

ADAM B. GREENBAUM, MD
Associate Professor of Medicine, Co-director
of the Emory Structural Heart and Valve
Center, Emory University Hospital, Atlanta,
Georgia, USA

ELLIOTT M. GROVES, MD, MEng, FACC,
FSCAI
Director, Structural Heart Interventions,
Assistant Professor, Division of Cardiology,
Department of Medicine, The University of
Illinois at Chicago, Jesse Brown VA Medical
Center, Chicago, Illinois, USA

PAUL GUEDENEY, MD
ACTION Coeur, Sorbonne Université, UMR_S
1166, Institut de Cardiologie (APHP), Hôpital
Pitié Salpêtrière, Paris, France

JONATHAN HILL, MA, MBChB, FRCP
King's College Hospital NHS Foundation
Trust, London, United Kingdom

GREGORY L. JUDSON, MD
Fellow, Division of Cardiology, University of
California, San Francisco, San Francisco,
California, USA

JAMES LEE, MD
Henry Ford Hospital, Detroit, Michigan, USA

VAIKOM S. MAHADEVAN, MD, FRCP,
FACC, FSCAI
Professor of Clinical Medicine, William W
Parmley Endowed Chair in Cardiology,
Director of Structural and Adult Congenital
Cardiac Interventions, Associate Chief of
Interventional Cardiology, Division of

Cardiology, University of California, San Francisco, San Francisco, California, USA

MOHAMMAD K. MOJADIDI, MD, FACP, FACC
Invasive Cardiologist, Assistant Professor, Division of Cardiology, Department of Medicine, Virginia Commonwealth University, Richmond, Virginia, USA

WILLIAM O'NEILL, MD
Medical Director, Center for Structural Heart Disease, Henry Ford Hospital, Detroit, Michigan, USA

LEONIDAS PALAIODIMOS, MD, MSc
Assistant Professor, Department of Medicine, Division of Hospital Medicine, Montefiore Medical Center, Albert Einstein College of Medicine, Bronx, New York, USA

DAVID A. POWER, MBBCh
The Zena and Michael A. Wiener Cardiovascular Institute, Icahn School of Medicine at Mount Sinai, New York, New York, USA

LENNART VAN GILS, MD, PhD
Research Fellow, Department of Interventional Cardiology, Thoraxcenter, Erasmus MC, Rotterdam, The Netherlands

NICOLAS M. VAN MIEGHEM, MD, PhD
Associate Professor, Department of Interventional Cardiology, Thoraxcenter, Erasmus MC, Rotterdam, The Netherlands

PEDRO VILLABLANCA, MD
Henry Ford Hospital, Detroit, Michigan, USA

DEE DEE WANG, MD
Henry Ford Hospital, Detroit, Michigan, USA

JULIAN YEOH, B.Pharm, MBBS, FRACP
King's College Hospital NHS Foundation Trust, London, United Kingdom

MARY RODRIGUEZ ZICCARDI, MD
Fellow of Cardiovascular Diseases, Division of Cardiology, Department of Medicine, The University of Illinois at Chicago, Chicago, Illinois, USA

CONTENTS

moderate to severe PPM. The outcomes for patients with larger effective orifice areas and lower gradients are better than for patients with PPM. With the advent of valve-in-valve TAVR, a degenerated surgical bioprosthesis can be treated with a percutaneous approach. However, the issue of PPM cannot be overcome by simply implanting a new valve. The technique of bioprosthetic valve fracture was therefore developed. This allows for implantation of a fully expanded transcatheter valve and results in a large effective orifice.

 Video content accompanies this article at http://www.interventional.theclinics.com.

Mitral valve disease becomes more prevalent as the population ages. As the number of percutaneous mitral valve interventions expands, obscure clinical scenarios may emerge and challenge conventional treatment algorithms. Strategies for dealing with complex repairs build on prior experience in mitral perivalvular leak repair. Cases using nitinol- and expanded polytetrafluoroethylene-based devices are used to treat mitral regurgitation in cases of focal mitral perforations and leaks between previously placed mitral valve edge-to-edge devices. This review discusses risks and benefits of performing such complex mitral repairs and informs clinicians of the strengths of weaknesses of different occluder devices in the mitral position.

Multiple transcatheter heart valve iterations have created an interesting range of options with which to perform transcatheter aortic valve replacement. The Lotus valve has several attractive features. The ability to eradicate even mild paravalvular leak mirrors the outcomes of surgical aortic valve replacement. New design iterations of the Lotus valve and refined sizing algorithms may help mitigate the need for permanent pacemaker implantation and consolidate its best-in-class results in terms of paravalvular leak. Ongoing trials should help define the safety and efficacy of the Lotus transcatheter heart valve in contemporary practice.

Conduction disturbances following TAVR are a common occurrence given the proximity of the various conduction system tissues, including the AV node, His-bundle, and bundle branches to the left ventricular outflow tract and aortic root. Impairment of these conduction system abnormalities may necessitate permanent pacemaker implantation, which increases morbidity and mortality, as well as length of stay, for the patient. The incidence, mechanisms, and predictors of conduction abnormalities and treatment options are discussed in this up-to-date review of the topic.

Intravascular lithotripsy facilitates percutaneous coronary intervention of lesions with severe calcification by using high-pressure ultrasonic energy. It is the newest adjunctive tool for calcium modification and is showing promise as its users gather more experience and it becomes readily available worldwide. This article reviews intravascular lithotripsy technology, the evidence in the literature, and the advantages and disadvantages compared with other forms of calcium modification, and discusses its role in specific subsets of coronary lesions. It concludes with a discussion about the future direction of research involving this new technology as its role within percutaneous cardiac procedures becomes more defined.

HOT TOPICS IN INTERVENTIONAL CARDIOLOGY

RELATED SERIES

Cardiology Clinics
Cardiac Electrophysiology Clinics
Heart Failure Clinics

THE CLINICS ARE NOW AVAILABLE ONLINE!

Access your subscription at:
www.theclinics.com

Pharmacodynamics During Transition Between Platelet P2Y$_{12}$ Inhibiting Therapies

Piera Capranzano, MD, PhD[a],*, Bruno Francaviglia, MD[a],
Dominick J. Angiolillo, MD, PhD[b]

KEYWORDS

- P2Y$_{12}$ inhibitors • Switching • Clopidogrel • Cangrelor • Prasugrel • Ticagrelor • Deescalation
- Escalation

KEY POINTS

- Several pharmacodynamic studies assessing the impact of switching between P2Y$_{12}$ inhibitors on platelet reactivity profiles have set the basis for defining optimal switching modalities.
- Escalation from the less (ie, clopidogrel) to the more potent (ie, prasugrel or ticagrelor) oral P2Y$_{12}$ inhibitors is associated with increased platelet inhibition without pharmacodynamic drug-drug interaction.
- De-escalation from the more to the less potent oral P2Y$_{12}$ inhibitors is associated with decreased platelet inhibition, with the potential for drug-drug interactions occurring with interclass (ie, from ticagrelor to clopidogrel) but not intraclass (ie, from prasugrel to clopidogrel) switching.
- When transitioning from cangrelor to an oral P2Y$_{12}$ inhibitor, prasugrel and clopidogrel should be given at the end of infusion to avoid a drug-drug interaction, whereas ticagrelor can be administered at any time (before, during, or end) without concerns for drug-drug interactions.

Dual antiplatelet therapy (DAPT) with aspirin plus an antagonist of the P2Y$_{12}$ receptor (ie, P2Y$_{12}$ inhibitor) is the mainstay treatment for the prevention of thrombotic complications after an acute coronary syndrome (ACS) and/or percutaneous coronary intervention (PCI).[1,2] The oral P2Y$_{12}$ inhibitors currently recommended in clinical practice comprise clopidogrel, prasugrel, and ticagrelor. Among the P2Y$_{12}$ inhibitors, cangrelor is the only intravenous agent. These antiplatelet drugs differ in pharmacodynamic and clinical profiles.[3] The availability of different P2Y$_{12}$ inhibitors may prompt the decision to switch therapies for several factors, including clinical presentation, bleeding risk, occurrence of an adverse event, side effects, and costs.[4,5] Several pharmacodynamic studies have been performed to assess the impact of switching on profiles of platelet reactivity and to define the optimal strategy to change between therapies, with the goal of avoiding the risk of having an inadequate platelet inhibition due to potential drug-drug interactions (DDI) occurring during the drug-overlapping phase.[6]

Disclosures: P. Capranzano and B. Francaviglia declare no conflicts of interest. D.J. Angiolillo declares that he has received consulting fees or honoraria from Amgen, Aralez, AstraZeneca, Bayer, Biosensors, Boehringer Ingelheim, Bristol-Myers Squibb, Chiesi, Daiichi-Sankyo, Eli Lilly, Haemonetics, Janssen, Merck, PLx Pharma, PhaseBio, Pfizer, Sanofi, and The Medicines Company and has received payments for participation in review activities from Celo-Nova and St Jude Medical. D.J. Angiolillo also declares that his institution has received research grants from Amgen, AstraZeneca, Bayer, Biosensors, CeloNova, CSL Behring, Daiichi-Sankyo, Eisai, Eli Lilly, Gilead, Idorsia, Janssen, Matsutani Chemical Industry Co., Merck, Novartis, Osprey Medical, and Renal Guard Solutions.
[a] Division of Cardiology, CAST Policlinico Hospital, University of Catania, S. Sofia n. 78, Catania 95123, Italy;
[b] Division of Cardiology, University of Florida College of Medicine, ACC Building 5th floor, 655 West 8th Street, Jacksonville, FL 32209, USA
* Corresponding author. Cardiology Division, CAST Policlinico Hospital, University of Catania, S. Sofia n. 78, Catania 95123, Italy.
E-mail address: pcapranzano@gmail.com

Intervent Cardiol Clin 8 (2019) 321–340
https://doi.org/10.1016/j.iccl.2019.05.001
2211-7458/19/© 2019 Elsevier Inc. All rights reserved.

This article provides an overview of pharmacodynamic studies assessing the switching between $P2Y_{12}$ inhibitors and recommendations on switching modalities based on these findings.

PHARMACOLOGIC DIFFERENCES BETWEEN $P2Y_{12}$ INHIBITORS

Key pharmacologic differences between $P2Y_{12}$ inhibitors that should be considered in assessing pharmacodynamic effects and the optimal strategy of switching therapies include the site and mechanism of $P2Y_{12}$ receptor binding; drug half-life; the speeds of onset and offset of pharmacodynamic effects; and the degree of platelet inhibition.[4–6]

Clopidogrel and prasugrel belong to the thienopyridine class and are both prodrugs that require metabolic activation through the hepatic cytochrome P450 (CYP) system to exert their antiplatelet effects.[7] Although the active metabolites of the 2 thienopyridines are equipotent, prasugrel has a far more efficient metabolism compared with clopidogrel, resulting in greater plasma levels of its active metabolites, which in turn translates into faster onset of action (2–8 hours vs 30 minutes–4 hours, respectively) and enhanced antiplatelet effects.[8] The thienopyridines' active metabolites occupy the adenosine diphosphate (ADP)-binding site on the $P2Y_{12}$ receptor, and this binding is irreversible, which renders the receptor nonfunctional for the platelet's life span. Because of this irreversible binding, the platelet reactivity recovery time to baseline after drug discontinuation approximates the life of platelets, that is, 7 to 10 days after prasugrel and 5 to 7 days after clopidogrel discontinuation.[9] The speed of complete offset of antiplatelet effect is longer for prasugrel compared with clopidogrel because of the enhanced level of platelet inhibition achieved with prasugrel. Finally, the active metabolite of clopidogrel is unstable, has a very short half-life (≈ 30 minutes), and is rapidly eliminated from the circulation if it does not bind to the $P2Y_{12}$ receptor.[7] The active metabolite of prasugrel is more stable than that of clopidogrel, but plasma levels decrease rapidly because of extensive extravascular distribution, resulting in a half-life of 30 to 60 minutes, after which levels detectable in the circulation (despite their long elimination half-life of 2–15 hours) may be insufficient to achieve effective $P2Y_{12}$ blockade.[7]

On the contrary from thienopyridines, ticagrelor is an oral cyclopentyl-triazolopyrimidine, which binds reversibly to the $P2Y_{12}$ receptor at a site that is distinct from the ADP-binding site.[10] It is a direct-acting agent that does not

require metabolic activation, but $\approx 30\%$ of its antiplatelet effect derives from an active metabolite (ARC124910XX) generated through CYP3A4/5 enzymes and with pharmacologic properties similar to those of the parent compound. Ticagrelor provides more prompt, potent, and predictable platelet inhibitory effects compared with clopidogrel.[11] A twice-daily dosing of ticagrelor is required because of its reversible receptor binding and a half-life of 8 to 12 hours. Despite being a reversibly acting agent with a relatively short half-life, ticagrelor's effects may persist for several days after drug discontinuation, with an offset of antiplatelet effect faster (3–5 days) compared with thienopyridines.[11] These observations are important to consider when switching from ticagrelor to a thienopyridine, given that if these latter agents are administered too early after discontinuation of ticagrelor (while the drug still occupies the receptor), the thienopyridine active metabolites will not be able to bind to the receptor and will thus be eliminated before the decline of the ticagrelor effect.[4–6]

Cangrelor is an intravenous adenosine triphosphate analogue that directly and reversibly inhibits ADP binding to the $P2Y_{12}$ receptor in a dose-dependent manner, achieving high levels of receptor occupancy and immediate (≈ 2 min) potent platelet inhibition after a bolus dose.[12] Enhanced platelet inhibition is provided by cangrelor even in patients treated with the more potent oral $P2Y_{12}$ inhibitors.[13,14] Cangrelor has a very short plasma half-life (3–6 minutes) allowing for a rapid (≈ 60 minutes) recovery of platelet function after its discontinuation.[12] The rapid offset of action, combined with a short half-life of thienopyridine active metabolites, implies that optimal timing is required to administer these latter agents after cangrelor infusion in order to allow the receptors to be unoccupied before the thienopyridine active metabolites are eliminated from the circulation.[4–6] The longer half-life of ticagrelor (and its major metabolite) makes it more versatile for use when switching from cangrelor to an oral $P2Y_{12}$ inhibitor.

DEFINITIONS OF TYPES OF SWITCHING

This section provides uniform definitions proposed by a focused expert consensus group to describe the type of switching based on the pharmacodynamic effects or class of $P2Y_{12}$ inhibitors interchanged and to standardize the timing of switching from the index ACS/PCI that led to the initiation of the $P2Y_{12}$ inhibitor.[15]

Switching Between Oral P2Y$_{12}$ Inhibitors

Prasugrel and ticagrelor provide enhanced pharmacodynamic effects compared with clopidogrel.[12] Therefore, switching from a less (ie, clopidogrel) to a more potent (ie, prasugrel or ticagrelor) P2Y$_{12}$ inhibitor results in an increase in platelet inhibition and is defined as "escalation." Vice versa, switching from a more potent to a less potent agent (ie, prasugrel or ticagrelor to clopidogrel) leads to less P2Y$_{12}$ inhibition and is defined as "deescalation." Although studies comparing the pharmacodynamic effects of prasugrel versus ticagrelor, defined as "change" (due to different class of agents), have provided inconsistent findings, the overall levels of P2Y$_{12}$ inhibition can be considered similar between these agents.[16] Such systematic terminology of switching modalities between oral P2Y$_{12}$ inhibitors (escalation, deescalation, and change) should be considered only when referring to the pharmacodynamic effects associated with the specific switching and should not imply any correlation with clinical efficacy or safety outcomes.

Switching between P2Y$_{12}$ inhibitors has also been classified according to the drug class. The P2Y$_{12}$ inhibitors belong to the thienopyridine (ie, clopidogrel or prasugrel) and cyclopentyl-triazolopyrimidine (ie, ticagrelor) families. The switching between drugs from the same or different class is defined as "intraclass" or "interclass," respectively.[15] A DDI is most likely to occur with an interclass switching. However, with escalation, no DDI have been described regardless of the switched drug classes. On the contrary, a DDI may occur with deescalation, especially with interclass switching from ticagrelor to clopidogrel. Finally, a DDI has been suggested with the interclass change switching from ticagrelor to prasugrel but not from prasugrel to ticagrelor.[15]

Oral P2Y$_{12}$ inhibitors can be switched at any time from the index event that led to initiation of these drugs. Because the thrombotic risk varies over time after an ACS/PCI, being highest in the first month, the timing of switching from the index event has an impact on the pharmacodynamic intensity of the switching strategy. In particular, different recommendations on how to switch therapies have been given for the early (within 30 days) and late (after 30 days) phases after the index event.[15]

Switching Between Intravenous and Oral P2Y$_{12}$ Inhibitors

Switching from an intravenous to an oral agent is defined as "transition," because cangrelor is used to achieve more rapid and potent platelet inhibition than the oral agents during the peri-PCI period and then it is necessary to shift to an oral P2Y$_{12}$ inhibitor for sustained, chronic antiplatelet effects after PCI.[15]

Switching from an oral P2Y$_{12}$ inhibitor to cangrelor is defined as "bridging," as it may occur in the peri-operative period, in order to maintain adequate level of platelet inhibition after interruption of an oral P2Y$_{12}$ inhibitor.[15] Although cangrelor is approved for use in patients who have not received an oral P2Y$_{12}$ inhibitor before PCI, it can be used on top of oral P2Y$_{12}$ inhibitors to bridge the gap in platelet inhibition associated with oral agents at the time of PCI, when an immediate effective antiplatelet effect is desired.

PHARMACODYNAMIC DATA AND STRATEGIES FOR SWITCHING BETWEEN ORAL P2Y$_{12}$ INHIBITORS

Data from available pharmacodynamic studies on escalation, deescalation, and change suggested recommendations on how to switch between oral P2Y$_{12}$ inhibitors if needed are described in this section. Switching modalities, depicted in **Fig. 1**, have been defined in a recent International Expert Consensus document on Switching Platelet P2Y$_{12}$ Receptor-Inhibiting Therapies[15] and have been also supported by the 2017 European Guidelines focusing on DAPT in coronary artery disease.[1] The American guidelines do not provide any specific recommendations on switching.[2,17]

Switching from Clopidogrel to Prasugrel or Ticagrelor (Escalation)

Pharmacodynamic studies that provide insights into levels of platelet inhibition associated with escalation from clopidogrel to prasugrel or ticagrelor can be grouped into 5 categories (**Tables 1–5**): (1) those comparing platelet reactivity while on clopidogrel (standard or high-dose regimens) versus prasugrel or ticagrelor with a crossover design[18–21]; (2) those assessing the pharmacodynamic effect of escalation in patients with high platelet reactivity (HPR) on clopidogrel or with diabetes[22–26]; (3) studies comparing intraclass versus interclass switching from clopidogrel[27,28]; (4) those assessing the impact of an escalation strategy with the loading dose (LD) versus prasugrel or ticagrelor alone[29–34]; and (5) those comparing different modalities of escalation (ie, with or without an LD of prasugrel or ticagrelor).[35–38]

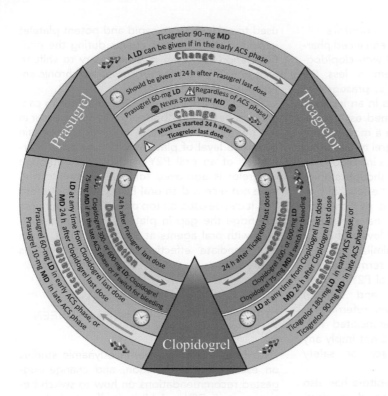

Fig. 1. Modalities for switching between oral P2Y$_{12}$ inhibitors. LD, loading dose; MD, maintenance dose.

Overall studies of the first 2 groups (see Tables 1 and 2) have shown that the escalation from clopidogrel to either prasugrel or ticagrelor leads to greater platelet inhibition regardless of clopidogrel responsiveness and dose regimens. In addition, studies of the third group (see Table 3) have shown that levels of platelet reactivity following escalation from clopidogrel are overall similar if switching to prasugrel or ticagrelor. The enhanced pharmacodynamic effects of prasugrel and ticagrelor compared with clopidogrel have translated into superior clinical efficacy among patients with ACS/PCI, at the expense of increased rates of major bleeding.[39,40] Escalation from clopidogrel to prasugrel or ticagrelor commonly occurs in patients with high-risk ACS undergoing PCI, who may have received pretreatment with clopidogrel at the time of admission. This escalation strategy is in accordance with guidelines suggesting that clopidogrel is a treatment option in patients with ACS only when prasugrel or ticagrelor are not available or are contraindicated.[1,2] However, only ticagrelor and clopidogrel are recommended in medically managed ACS, whereas prasugrel use is restricted only to patients undergoing PCI.[1] Another condition that can lead to escalation of P2Y$_{12}$ inhibition could be a thrombotic event occurring while on DAPT with aspirin and

clopidogrel. Finally, escalation of P2Y$_{12}$ inhibition could occur in patients with ACS initially treated with thrombolysis, during which clopidogrel is the P2Y$_{12}$ inhibitor of choice, and then switching to prasugrel or ticagrelor 48 hours after thrombolytic therapy can be achieved.

Studies belonging to the fourth category (see Table 4) have shown that platelet reactivity with prasugrel or ticagrelor LD was not different if those drugs were given on top of clopidogrel, 600 mg. Subanalyses of randomized data, available only for the escalation from clopidogrel to ticagrelor from the PLATO trial, showed that pretreatment with clopidogrel LD did not affect the safety and efficacy of ticagrelor versus clopidogrel.[40] Moreover, several registries have consistently shown no increase in major bleeding associated with switching from clopidogrel to prasugrel.[41,42]

Finally, the fifth category of studies (see Table 5) on escalation has shown that enhanced platelet inhibition levels following the switching from clopidogrel to prasugrel or ticagrelor are achieved more promptly after administration of an LD compared with an MD regimen. Based on these studies it has been suggested that escalation from clopidogrel to ticagrelor or prasugrel can be achieved with the LD or directly with the maintenance dose (MD) if this occurs

Table 1
Studies comparing platelets inhibition on clopidogrel versus prasugrel or ticagrelor with a crossover design

Study Name (Acronym)	Study Design	Study Population	Compared Arms	Main Pharmacodynamic Results
Wiviott et al,[18] 2007 (PRINCIPLE-TIMI 44)	Randomized, double-blind, double-dummy, crossover	Planned PCI (N = 201)	C 600/150 mg vs P 60/10 mg	Escalation: LTA IPA 45% on 150 mg C → 61% after 15 d on 10 mg P. Deescalation: IPA 61.9% on 10 mg P → 46.8% after 15 d on 150 mg C.
Montalescot et al,[19] 2010 (ACAPULCO)	Randomized, double-blind, crossover	UA/NSTEMI (N = 56)	From 900 mg C to C 150 mg vs P 10 mg	Escalation: LTA MPA 38.6% after 900 mg C → 28.9% after 15 d on 10 mg P. MPA 38.6% after 900 mg C → 38.2% after 15 d on 150 mg C → 25% after 15 d on 10 mg P. Deescalation: MPA 28.9% on 10 mg P → 42.5% after 15 d on 150 mg C.
Sardella et al,[20] 2012 (RESET GENE)	Randomized, open-label, crossover	Stable CAD with HPR undergoing PCI (N = 32)	C 150 mg vs P 10 mg	Escalation: MEA AUC 576 on C → 180.5 after 15 d on P 10 mg MEA AUC 380.5 on 150 mg C → 256 after 15 d on 10 mg P. Deescalation: AUC 180.5 after 15 on 10 mg P → 330 after 15 d on 150 mg C.
Gurbel et al,[21] 2010 (RESPOND)	Randomized, double-blind, double-dummy, crossover	Stable CAD (N = 98)	C 600/75 mg vs T 180/90 mg	Escalation: Nonresponder cohort: LTA MPA 59 ± 9% on C → 35 ± 11% 4 h after 180 mg T. Responder cohort: MPA 47 ± 15% on C → 32 ± 8%, 4 h after 180 mg T. Deescalation: Nonresponder cohort: MPA 36 ± 14% on T → 56 ± 9% 4 h after 600 mg C. Responder cohort: MPA 25 ± 11% on T → 45 ± 8% 4 h after 600 mg C.

Abbreviations: AUC, area under the curve; C, clopidogrel; CAD, coronary artery disease; HPR, high on-treatment platelet reactivity; IPA, inhibition of platelet aggregation; LTA, light transmission aggregometry; MEA, multiple electrode platelet aggregometry; MPA, maximal platelet aggregation; NSTEMI, non-ST elevation myocardial infarction; P, prasugrel; T, ticagrelor; UA, unstable angina.

Table 2
Studies assessing escalation in patients with on clopidogrel high on-treatment platelet reactivity or diabetics

Study Name, Acronym	Design	Population	Switching Type	Main Pharmacodynamic Results
Trenk et al,[22] 2012 (TRIGGER-PCI)	Randomized, parallel assignment, double-blind	Stable CAD with HPR undergoing PCI (N = 212)	From C to C 75 mg vs P 10 mg	Decrease in PRU with P compared with C. 176 (94.1%) patients with P reached a PRU ≤208.
Cuisset et al,[23] 2013	Prospective observational registry	NSTE-ACS with diabetes undergoing PCI (N = 107)	From C 600 mg to P 10 mg	PRI 47 ± 21% after 600 mg C → 31 ± 13% after 1 mo on 10 mg P.
Aradi et al,[24] 2014	Prospective observational registry	ACS undergoing PCI (N = 741) On clopidogrel HPR switched (n = 219)	From C to P 60/10 mg vs high-dose C	P 60/10 mg provided more potent platelet inhibition than the repeated 600 mg C LD. 86% of the P MD-treated patients remained below the HPR cut-point.
Mayer et al,[25] 2014 (ISAR-HPR)	Prospective observational registry	HPR patients undergoing PCI (N = 571)	From C 600 mg to P 60 mg	AU*min 651 (543–780) after 600 mg C → 156 (88–261) after 60 mg P.
Capranzano et al,[26] 2011	Prospective observational registry	Elderly patients with ACS undergoing PCI (N = 100) On clopidogrel HPR switched (n = 20)	From C 75 mg to P 10 mg	PRU mean 279.8 ± 45.1 on C → 171.7 ± 65.2 after 15 d on 5 mg P.

Abbreviations: AU*min, aggregation unit * minutes; C, clopidogrel; CAD, coronary artery disease; HPR, high on-treatment platelet reactivity; LD, loading dose; MD, maintenance dose; NSTE, non-ST elevation; P, prasugrel; PRU, P2Y$_{12}$ reaction units; T, ticagrelor.

Table 3
Studies comparing intraclass versus interclass switching from clopidogrel

Study Name, Acronym	Design	Population	Compared Arms	Main Pharmacodynamic Results
Rollini et al,[27] 2016	Prospective, randomized, parallel design, open-label	CAD (N = 110)	From C to P 60/10 mg vs T 180/90 mg	MPA 50.3±% on C→ 32 ± 6% 30 min after 60 mg P→ 18.8 ± 4% 2 h after 60 mg P→ 16.6 ± 2% 24 h after 60 mg P→ 28.6 ± 4% 1 wk after 60 mg P. MPA 50.2 ± 6% on C→ 42 ± 6% 30 min after 180 mg T→ 21.9 ± 4% 2 h after 180 mg T→ 18.9 ± 1.1% 24 h after 180 mg T (12 h after 90 mg T→ 34 ± 4% 1 wk after 180 mg T (12 h after 90 mg T). Platelet reactivity was similar between T and P
Alexopoulos et al,[28] 2012	Prospective, randomized, single-blind, crossover	ACS with on clopidogrel HPR (N = 44)	From C to P 10 mg vs T 90 mg	PRU 280.3 on C→ 90.8 after 15 d on 10 mg P→ 32.1 after 15 d on 90 mg T. PRU 277.4 on C→ 34.1 after 15 d on 90 mg T→ 111.4 after 15 d on 10 mg P. T provided higher platelet inhibition than P, with no differences in HPR rates.

Abbreviations: C, clopidogrel; CAD, coronary artery disease; HPR, high on-treatment platelet reactivity; MPA, maximal platelet aggregation; P, prasugrel; PRU, P2Y$_{12}$ reaction units; T, ticagrelor.

in the acute or in the late phase of ACS/PCI, respectively. Ticagrelor or prasugrel administration can occur at any time from the last LD or MD of clopidogrel, as no DDI or concerns of overdosing have been shown with escalation. Thus, in the acute phase, one should consider administering the LD as soon as possible if the objective is to achieve immediate and enhanced platelet inhibition (eg, in a patient with high-risk ACS undergoing PCI). Differently, if escalation occurs in the late phase, it is practical to administer the ticagrelor or prasugrel MD at the time of the next scheduled dose of P2Y$_{12}$ inhibiting therapy (ie, at about 24 hours from the last dose of clopidogrel).[15]

Switching from Prasugrel or Ticagrelor to Clopidogrel (Deescalation)

Several pharmacodynamic studies, including those comparing clopidogrel with the more potent oral PY$_{12}$ inhibitors (summarized in Table 1[18–21]) have shown that a deescalation strategy is associated with lower levels of platelet inhibition on clopidogrel, with increased rates of HPR (Table 6).[43–46] Based on these pharmacodynamic findings, deescalation should more commonly occur in patients with factors

associated with high bleeding risk requiring less potent platelet inhibition. In addition, the observation that the greatest antiischemic benefits of more potent P2Y$_{12}$ inhibitors are seen early, although most bleeding arise during chronic treatment with these drugs,[47,48] has set the rationale for deescalating P2Y$_{12}$ inhibition after the early high-ischemic risk phase of an ACS, regardless of the bleeding risk, with the goal of reducing bleeding while maximizing ischemic benefit. The reduced costs associated with the use of clopidogrel may also be a contributing factor to this strategy.

The clinical consequences of this latter deescalation strategy have been assessed in 2 randomized trials.[49,50] The TOPIC (Timing of Platelet Inhibition After Acute Coronary Syndrome) trial compared a group (n = 322) switching from prasugrel or ticagrelor to clopidogrel at 1 month after ACS (without guidance from platelet function testing or genetic testing) with a group (n = 323) conventionally treated with 1-year DAPT including prasugrel or ticagrelor.[49] In this study, the deescalation strategy compared with unchanged DAPT was associated with lower 1-year rates of the composite endpoint of cardiovascular death, urgent

Table 4
Impact of escalation versus prasugrel or ticagrelor alone

Study Name, Acronym	Design	Population	Compared Arms	Main Pharmacodynamic Results
Diodati et al,[29] 2013 (TRIPLET)	Randomized, double-blind, double-dummy, 3-arm, parallel, active-controlled	ACS undergoing planned PCI (N = 282)	P 60 mg only vs C 600 mg + P 60 or 30 mg (P was given 24 h after C)	PRU 57.9, 6 h after placebo/ 60 mg P. PRU 35.6, 6 h after 600 mg C/ 60 mg P. PRU 53.9, 6 h after C 600 mg/ 30 mg P.
Koul et al,[30] 2014	Prospective observational registry	STEMI undergoing PCI (N = 223)	Pre-H C only Or Pre-H C to P Or P only Or Pre-H C to T Or T only	PRI 79% after 600 mg C (pre-PCI)→ 74% after 60 mg P 60 (after PCI)→ 17% 1 d after PCI. PRI 64% after 600 mg C (pre-PCI)→ 53% after 180 mg T (after PCI)→ 29% 1 d after PCI. Platelet inhibition 1 d after PCI was similar between the 2 escalation groups vs P or T only.
Nührenberg et al,[31] 2013	Nonrandomized, observational	STEMI undergoing PCI (N = 47)	P 60 mg only vs Pre-H C + P 60-mg (pre-PCI)	PRU 10 (8–31) after 600 mg C+60 mg P. PRU 9 [6–60] after 60 mg P only. No differences in platelet inhibition 1 d after PCI between the escalation group vs P only.
Parodi et al,[32] 2014	Nonrandomized, observational	CAD undergoing PCI (N = 454)	P 60 mg only vs C 600 mg + P 60 mg (given 1 ± 2 d after C)	MPA 45 ± 18% in the escalation group vs 36 ± 17% in P only HPR group: MPA 72 ± 11% on C → 43 ± 16% on P.

| Lhermusier et al,[33] 2014 | Open-label, multicenter, nonrandomized observational | ACS with planned invasive strategy (N = 75) | P 60 mg only vs C 600 mg + P 60 mg | PRU 234 (164–267) after 600 mg C → 23 (5–71) 4 h after 60 mg P → 9 (5–47) at discharge on 10 mg P. PRU 23 [5–71] in the escalation group vs 54 [5–91] in the P only 4 h after P. |
| Hibbert et al,[34] 2014 (CAPITAL RELOAD) | Prospective, observational | STEMI (N = 52) | T 180 mg only vs C 600 mg + T 180 mg | PRU 252 (233–280) naive patients→220(82–269) 2 h after T 180 mg. PRU 255 (233–304) after C 600 mg →90 (5–205) 2 h after T 180 mg. The escalation group had lower PRU values from 2–48 h. |

Abbreviations: C, clopidogrel; CAD, coronary artery disease; HPR, high on-treatment platelet reactivity; MPA, maximal platelet aggregation; P, prasugrel; PRI, platelet reactivity index; PRU, P2Y$_{12}$ reaction units; STEMI, ST-elevation myocardial infarction; T, ticagrelor.

Table 5
Studies comparing different escalation modalities, with or without loading dose

Study Name, Acronym	Design	Population	Compared Arms	Main Pharmacodynamic Results
Payne et al,[35] 2008	Randomized, open-label, fixed sequence	Healthy subjects (N = 35)	From C 75 mg to P 60/10-mg vs P 10-mg	MPA 37% on C → 5% 1 h after 60 mg P. MPA 37% on C → 28% 1 h after 10 mg P.
Angiolillo et al,[36] 2010 (SWAP)	Randomized, double-blind, double-dummy, active-control	Prior ACS (30–330 d) (N = 139)	From C 75 mg to Placebo LD/C 75 mg vs P 60/10 mg vs Placebo LD/P 10 mg	MPA 60.2% on C 75 mg → 41.1% after 7 d on 10 mg P. MPA 55.5% on C 75 mg → 41% after 60 mg P+7 d of 10 mg P. MPA 53.8% on 75 mg C → 55% after 7 d on 75 mg C. At 2 h, P 60/10 mg resulted in higher platelet inhibition vs other regimens
Lhermusier et al,[37] 2014	Prospective, open-label, randomized	ACS (N = 48)	From C 600 mg to C 75 mg vs P 10 mg vs T 90 mg vs P 30/10 mg vs T 180/90 mg	PRU 143 (53–199) after 600 mg C → 111 (7–127) 4 h after 10 mg P → 97 (41–145), 24 h after P. PRU 122 (82–149) after 600 mg C → 7 (6–31), 4 h after 30 mg P → 27 (7–20) 24 h after initial P dose. PRU 146 (97–236) after 600 mg C → 12 (4–46), 4 h after 90 mg T → 9 (5–10), 24 h after T. PRU 92 (33–143) after 600 mg C → 4(2–6), 4 h after 180 mg T → 4 (3–5), 24 h after initial T dose.
Caiazzo et al,[38] 2014 (SHIFT-OVER)	Randomized, single-blind	ACS (N = 50)	From C to T 90 mg vs T 180 mg	AU 34.4 ± 1.3 on C → 17.6 ± 7.2, 2 h after 90 mg T. AU 41.7 ± 2 on C → 18.1 ± 6, 2 h after 180 mg T. No difference in aggregation between T 90 mg and T 180 mg

Abbreviations: AU, aggregation unit; C, clopidogrel; CAD, coronary artery disease; MPA, maximal platelet aggregation; P, prasugrel; PRU, P2Y$_{12}$ reaction units; T, ticagrelor.

Table 6
Pharmacodynamic studies on P2Y$_{12}$ inhibitor deescalation

Study Name, Acronym	Design	Population	Switching Type	Main Pharmacodynamic Results
Kerneis et al,[43] 2013	Prospective, observational registry	ACS (N = 31)	From P 10 mg to C 75 mg	MPA 21.01 ± 10.47% on 10 mg P → 43.84 ± 15.19% after 15 d on 75 mg C.
Deharo et al,[44] 2013 (POBA)	Prospective, observational	ACS with LPR (N = 20)	From P 10 mg to C 75 mg	PRI 7 ± 2% on P → 37.8 ± 15.6% after 1 mo on C
Pourdjabbar et al,[45] 2017 (CAPITAL OPTICROSS)	Prospective, randomized, open-label	ACS (N = 60)	From T to C 600/75 mg vs C 75 mg	PRU ~40 on T → 114 ± 73.1, 48 h after 600 mg C. PRU ~40 on T → 165.1 ± 70.5, 48 h after 75 mg C.
Franchi et al,[46] 2018 (SWAP-4)	Prospective, randomized, open-label	Stable CAD (N = 80)	From T 180/90 mg for 7 ± 2 to C 600/75 mg (24 h after last T) vs C 600/75 mg (12 h after last T) vs C 75 mg vs T 90 mg	Lower platelet inhibition in the deescalation groups vs continuing T. Similar platelet inhibition levels between C groups at 48 h. Lower platelet inhibition with C LD during the first 48 h. No differences in platelet inhibition between C LD groups (12 vs 24 h after T last dose)

Abbreviations: C, clopidogrel; LD, loading dose; LPR, low platelet reactivity; MPA, maximal platelet aggregation; P, prasugrel; PRI, platelet reactivity index; PRU, P2Y$_{12}$ reaction units.

revascularization, stroke, and bleeding defined by the Bleeding Academic Research Consortium (BARC) classification greater than or equal to 2. The study findings were driven by reductions in bleeding without increasing overall ischemic events.[49] The TROPICAL-ACS (Testing Responsiveness To Platelet Inhibition On Chronic Antiplatelet Treatment For Acute Coronary Syndromes) trial compared a group (n = 1304) treated with a deescalation strategy guided by platelet function testing (prasugrel for 1 week after ACS followed by 1-week clopidogrel and a subsequent platelet function testing–guided maintenance therapy with clopidogrel or prasugrel from day 14 after hospital discharge) with a group (n = 1306) receiving a conventional, nonguided 12-month treatment with prasugrel.[50] In this study, guided deescalation of antiplatelet treatment was noninferior to standard treatment with prasugrel at 1 year after PCI in terms of net clinical benefit (composite of cardiovascular death, myocardial infarction, stroke, or BARC $\geq$2 bleeding).[50] Although there were no differences in bleeding between groups (likely due to the fact that many patients in the guided group need to switch back to prasugrel), there was no increase in ischemic events with guided deescalation in this high-risk group of patients. With regard to the impact of platelet reactivity levels at the time of switching on the treatment effect of deescalation, in the TOPIC trial the switched DAPT was superior regardless of initial platelet reactivity, although the benefit was greater in patients with low on-treatment platelet reactivity.[51] This enhanced benefit of DAPT deescalation could be explained by the fact that low on-treatment platelet reactivity has emerged as the strongest independent predictor of bleeding in the platelet function analysis from the TROPICAL-ACS trial.[52]

Despite the favorable clinical profile of deescalation shown in the TOPIC and TROPICAL-ACS trials, these studies were not powered to detect differences in ischemic outcomes, and no definitive conclusions can be drawn on the clinical efficacy of the $P2Y_{12}$ deescalation strategy in the late ACS phase. For this reason, the 2018 European guidelines provide a Class IIb recommendation in that $P2Y_{12}$ inhibitors deescalation guided by platelet function testing may be considered as an alternative DAPT strategy, especially for patients with ACS deemed unsuitable for a 12-month potent platelet inhibition, such as those at high bleeding risk.[53] There are several ongoing trials using genetic testing as a strategy to deescalate antiplatelet therapy.[54] The topic of deescalation and guidance on how to integrate platelet function and genetic testing has been recently reported in an updated international consensus document.[55]

Although a decrease in platelet inhibition is anticipated with deescalation, it is relevant to define the strategy associated with a less abrupt increase in platelet reactivity and to rule out a DDI. Only 2 pharmacodynamic studies have compared different deescalation strategies (ie, dosing and timing of clopidogrel) and have focused on the interclass switching from ticagrelor to clopidogrel (see **Table 6**).[45,46] The CAPITAL OPTI-CROSS study found that deescalating with a clopidogrel LD was associated with reduced rates of HPR at 48 hours, with no differences between groups after 72 hours, compared with switching directly to clopidogrel with an MD.[45] Consistently with these findings, the switching antiplatelet therapy (SWAP)-4 randomized study showed that switching from ticagrelor to clopidogrel with an LD was associated with enhanced platelet inhibition during the first 48 hours compared with switching directly to a clopidogrel MD regimen, with no pharmacodynamic differences according to the timing of LD administration after the last dose of ticagrelor (ie, 12 vs 24 hours).[46] In addition, the SWAP-4 study showed that switching from ticagrelor to clopidogrel was associated with pharmacodynamic profiles that suggest a DDI, as levels of platelet reactivity after switching were higher compared with values observed at baseline while on clopidogrel therapy. These effects were mitigated with the use of a clopidogrel LD compared with an MD.[46] The more favorable pharmacodynamic profile of the switching modality with a clopidogrel LD versus MD can be explained by the fact that ticagrelor has a relatively fast offset of action, requiring a more rapid achievement of clopidogrel's full therapeutic effect, avoiding an abrupt increase in platelet reactivity after deescalation. For this reason, when deescalating from ticagrelor, the use of a clopidogrel LD is recommended. Deescalation using a clopidogrel MD may be considered only when the switching occurs because of an active bleeding.

No studies have assessed the pharmacodynamic effect of deescalating from prasugrel with or without a clopidogrel LD, but it has been reasonably suggested to switch directly with a clopidogrel MD, which can allow a full antiplatelet effect of clopidogrel to eventually be reached during the prolonged offset of prasugrel. However, the use of a clopidogrel LD should be considered if deescalation from prasugrel occurs in the early ACS phase, when platelet recovery after prasugrel discontinuation may be shorter, leading to a window of a lower platelet inhibition before clopidogrel reaches its full effects.[15]

Switching Between Prasugrel and Ticagrelor (Change)

Based on studies comparing the antiplatelet effect of ticagrelor versus prasugrel, no meaningful differences in levels of platelet inhibition are expected when switching between these 2 agents.[16] Indeed, although escalation and deescalation occur in scenarios where more or less pronounced platelet inhibition, respectively, is required, reasons for change between the newer generation P2Y$_{12}$ inhibitors may include side effects, the development of contraindications, costs, and compliance issues. In clinical practice, ticagrelor-related dyspnea is among the main reasons prompting the change from ticagrelor to prasugrel.[41,42]

There are limited studies of the pharmacodynamic effects associated with a change between prasugrel and ticagrelor.[56,57] The pharmacodynamic effects of switching from ticagrelor to prasugrel was investigated in the SWAP-2 study, in which patients were randomly assigned to continue ticagrelor or to switch to prasugrel with or without a 60 mg LD given 12 hours after the last ticagrelor MD.[56] In this study, platelet reactivity was higher in patients treated with prasugrel (combined groups) compared with those treated with ticagrelor at 7 days, not meeting the noninferiority primary endpoint, although there was no difference in rates of HPR between groups. At 24 hours and up to 48 hours after the switch, platelet reactivity increased in patients switched to prasugrel compared with preswitch levels. However, the increase in platelet reactivity after switching, which suggests a DDI, was mitigated by administration of a prasugrel LD.[56] The mechanisms for these findings might likely be the result of prolonged binding of ticagrelor to the P2Y$_{12}$ receptor after plasma levels have decreased, which may potentially impede the active metabolites of thienopyridines to access their binding site before being eliminated from the circulation. Based on the SWAP-2 results it has been suggested that change from ticagrelor to prasugrel should be achieved by starting always with a prasugrel 60 mg LD, regardless of the timing from the index event that required initiation of the P2Y$_{12}$ inhibitor, in order to partially overcome the DDI. In addition, switching to prasugrel at a later time after MD (ie, after 24 hours) should limit increases in platelet reactivity, by providing more time for

P2Y$_{12}$ receptor blockade by ticagrelor to decline.[15]

The pharmacodynamic effects of switching from prasugrel to ticagrelor were investigated in the SWAP-3 study. This study demonstrated that changing to ticagrelor was associated with transient reductions in platelet reactivity, observed as early as 2 hours and up to 48 hours after switching.[57] No differences were observed between switching with ticagrelor 180 mg LD or 90 mg MD. Thus, in the SWAP-3 study, no DDI has been shown when changing from prasugrel to ticagrelor, allowing a switch directly with a ticagrelor MD (90 mg), which should be started at the time of the next scheduled dose.[57] However, the administration of a ticagrelor LD 24 hours after prasugrel last dose should be considered when change from prasugrel to ticagrelor occurs in the acute phase of an ACS.[15]

SWITCHING BETWEEN CANGRELOR AND ORAL P2Y$_{12}$ INHIBITORS

Cangrelor has been approved for use during PCI based on a large randomized trial showing that the transition from cangrelor to clopidogrel versus clopidogrel was associated with reduced ischemic events, with no significant increase in severe bleeding.[58] The optimal strategy for transitioning from cangrelor to the oral P2Y$_{12}$ inhibitors is key to achieve sustained P2Y$_{12}$ inhibition after PCI and has been investigated in several pharmacodynamic studies (**Table 7**).[59–65]

The transition from cangrelor to clopidogrel has been associated with an impaired antiplatelet effect when clopidogrel is administered during cangrelor infusion.[59,60] This is because the active metabolite of clopidogrel is eliminated before receptors become unoccupied by cangrelor and thus available for binding. Because cangrelor has a rapid offset of action, the antiplatelet effects of clopidogrel are not diminished when it is administered at the end of cangrelor infusion, which is the recommended strategy when transitioning from cangrelor to clopidogrel and the strategy on which cangrelor was approved for clinical practice.

The administration of prasugrel during cangrelor infusion is associated with recovery of platelet reactivity, which is attenuated when prasugrel is administered 30 minutes before cangrelor infusion is stopped.[63] However, a study showed that a 60 mg LD of prasugrel given at the start of a 2-hour infusion of cangrelor was associated with sufficient platelet inhibition at 1 hour after stopping cangrelor.[64] Despite these results, until additional data are available that

Table 7
Studies on transition from cangrelor to oral P2Y$_{12}$ inhibitors

Study Name, Acronym	Design	Population	Assessed Arms	Main Pharmacodynamic Results
Steinhubl et al,[59] 2008	Randomized, open-label	Healthy volunteers (N = 20)	C 600 mg and Cang simultaneously vs C 600 mg alone vs C 600 mg given at the end of Cang infusion	Complete platelet inhibition during Cang infusion. C at the end of Cang infusion and alone: max inhibition 3 h and 2 h after C, respectively. C and Cang simultaneously: platelet reactivity similar to baseline (no antiplatelet therapy) at all time points.
Schneider et al,[60] 2015	Prospective not randomized	Stable CAD (N = 12)	C 600 mg 0.5 h prior stop Cang vs C 600 mg 1 h prior stop Cang vs C 600 mg at the end of Cang	LTA MPA ≤2% during Cang infusion. MPA 1 h after stop Cang infusion: 56 ± 9% with C at the end of infusion, 56 ± 17% with C 30 min prior stop infusion, 65 ± 10% with C 1 h prior stop infusion.
Angiolillo et al,[61] 2012	Predefined substudy of CHAMPION-PCI and CHAMPION-PLATFORM randomized trials	CAD undergoing PCI (N = 167)	Cang + C vs placebo/C	PRU 93.5 on Cang → ~240 6–12 h after stopping infusions and administering C. Postinfusion PRU was not significantly different between Cang + C vs placebo + C.
Schneider et al,[62] 2014	Prospective not randomized	Stable CAD (N = 12)	Cang + T 180 mg at 0.5 h after Cang Or Cang + T 180 mg at 1.25 h after Cang Or T given 12 h before Cang infusion	Switching from Cang to T (0.5 h): LTA MPA: 3.5 ± 1.9% on Cang→16 ± 15%, 30 min after stopping infusion. Switching from Cang to T (1.25 h): LTA MPA: 1.2 ± 1.9% on Cang → 21 ± 17%, 30 min after stopping infusion. Switching from T to Cang: LTA MPA: 12 ± 9% on T→1.5 ± 1.9 during Cang infusion.

Study	Study design	Population	Intervention	Findings
Schneider et al,[63] 2015	Prospective not randomized	Stable CAD (N = 15)	Cang infusion + P 60 mg at 1 h, 1.5 h, 2 h, or 2.5 h Or P given 24 h before Cang infusion	Switching from Cang to P: LTA MPA: <4% on Cang → 41% 30 min after stopping infusion when P administered 30 before infusion stop; ~60%, 30 min after stopping infusion when P administered 1 before infusion stop or at the end of infusion. Switching from P to Cang: LTA MPA: <5% on P → <5%, during Cang infusion.
Hochholzer et al,[64] 2017	Prospective, randomized, open-label	CAD undergoing PCI (n = 110)	Transition from Cang to P 60 mg simultaneously vs T 180 mg simultaneously vs C 600 mg at the end of infusion	Platelet reactivity (median): 94 AU on Cang → 212 on C, 154 on P, 81 on T, at 1 h after stopping infusion. HPR rates at 1 h after stopping Cang: 35% on C; 6.7% on P; 4.4% on T.
Franchi et al,[65] 2019, CANTIC	Prospective, randomized, double-blind, placebo-controlled	STEMI patients undergoing primary PCI	Cang + T (crushed) simultaneously vs Placebo infusion/T crushed	PRU 63 (32–93) with Cang + T vs 214 (183–245) with T alone 30 min after starting therapy. No differences in platelet reactivity between groups after discontinuation of Cang/placebo infusion.

Abbreviations: AU, aggregation units per min; C, clopidogrel; CAD, coronary artery disease; Cang, cangrelor; HPR, high platelets reactivity; LTA, light transmission aggregometry; MPA, maximal platelet aggregation; P, prasugrel; PRU, P2Y$_{12}$ reaction units; STEMI, ST-elevation myocardial infarction; T, ticagrelor.

confirms these findings, it has been prudently suggested to administer prasugrel at the end of cangrelor infusion, in order to prevent the transient gap in platelet inhibition. Although cangrelor is approved for use in $P2Y_{12}$ inhibitors-naïve patients before PCI, for those patients who have been pretreated with a thienopyridine, if the pretreatment time was shortly before the initiation of cangrelor, or is not known, a thienopyridine reloading at the end of cangrelor infusion should be considered.[15]

During the transition from cangrelor to ticagrelor, a nonsignificant increase in platelet reactivity was observed during the first hour after cangrelor was stopped, which seemed to be attenuated with earlier administration of ticagrelor.[62] Thus, differently from thienopyridines, no interaction was shown for the transition from cangrelor to ticagrelor, due to the longer half-life of the latter. For this reason, ticagrelor can be given before, during, or at the end of the cangrelor infusion, although the expert consensus suggested that earlier administration of ticagrelor (eg, at the time of PCI) should be considered over administration at the end of cangrelor infusion to minimize the potential gap in platelet inhibition during the transition phase. The recent CANTIC (the Platelet Inhibition with CANgrelor and Crushed TICagrelor in STEMI Patients Undergoing Primary Percutaneous Coronary Intervention) randomized pharmacodynamic study has shown that in patients undergoing primary PCI for ST-elevation myocardial infarction (STEMI), the concomitant administration of crushed ticagrelor and cangrelor was more effective than crushed ticagrelor alone in reducing platelet reactivity at 5 minutes after the cangrelor bolus and over the 2 hours of the cangrelor infusion, with no differences in platelet inhibition after the cangrelor infusion was discontinued.[65] Therefore, this study suggested that transition from cangrelor to ticagrelor, with this latter drug given at the start of the infusion, represents an effective strategy to bridge the gap in platelet inhibition associated with the use of only ticagrelor, without any apparent DDI between the 2 drugs. Considering that effective $P2Y_{12}$ inhibition reached during PCI for STEMI could be beneficial,[66] the use of cangrelor as a bridge to oral $P2Y_{12}$ inhibitors in the setting of STEMI might potentially improve outcomes. However, studies assessing the clinical safety and efficacy of cangrelor versus more potent oral $P2Y_{12}$ inhibitors in the setting of STEMI are lacking.

With regard to bridging from an oral $P2Y_{12}$ inhibitor to cangrelor in the presurgical setting, the infusion of cangrelor can be started 3 to 4 days after prasugrel and 2 to 3 days after clopidogrel or ticagrelor discontinuations, in order to avoid unnecessary infusion during the time in which adequate platelet inhibition may still persist after oral $P2Y_{12}$ inhibitors interruption. In a pharmacodynamic randomized trial performed among patients who discontinue $P2Y_{12}$ inhibitors before cardiac surgery, bridging with cangrelor consistently achieved and maintained platelet inhibition at levels known to be associated with a low thrombotic risk, with no differences in surgery-related bleeding compared with placebo.[67] However, clinical safety and efficacy associated with cangrelor bridging before surgery remain to be confirmed in larger studies. Recommendations for considering bridging have been recently summarized in a national expert collaborative document.[68]

SUMMARY

Pharmacologic, clinical, and cost differences between platelet $P2Y_{12}$ inhibitors have enabled physicians to consider switching between agents. Although robust evidence for clinical outcomes with specific switching strategies are lacking, several pharmacodynamic studies have provided the basis for defining optimal switching strategies that can support physician decision-making in specific clinical settings where a switch from one $P2Y_{12}$ inhibitor to another is needed. In summary, escalation from the less to the more potent oral $P2Y_{12}$ inhibitors is associated with increased platelet inhibition without pharmacodynamic DDI, translating in no clinical safety issues of this strategy based on available evidence. Differently, deescalation of oral $P2Y_{12}$ inhibitors is associated with decreased platelet inhibition and with DDI if this occurs between different classes of agents, which can be partially mitigated by switching with a clopidogrel LD. Thus, despite the rationale and potential practical advantages of $P2Y_{12}$ deescalation in the late ACS phase have fueled particular interest, further clinical investigations are needed before it can be routinely applied. With regard to the change between the 2 more potent $P2Y_{12}$ inhibitors, although no DDI have been shown for the switching from prasugrel to ticagrelor, change from ticagrelor to prasugrel has been associated with significant increase in platelet reactivity that can be mitigated by using a prasugrel LD, which also suggests that changing should be done only when it is deemed clinically necessary. Finally, transition from cangrelor to oral $P2Y_{12}$ inhibitors is associated with sustained platelet inhibition when prasugrel and clopidogrel were given at the end of cangrelor infusion. Differently, platelet reactivity after cangrelor infusion is not affected by the timing of ticagrelor administration, despite more optimal inhibition being observed when ticagrelor is given earlier during infusion. Future studies are warranted to better clarify the role of a transition from cangrelor to more potent oral P2Y$_{12}$ inhibitors in different clinical scenarios. Moreover, further investigations are needed to assess safety and efficacy of bridging from P2Y$_{12}$ inhibitors to cangrelor in the presurgical period.

REFERENCES

1. Valgimigli M, Bueno H, Byrne RA, et al, ESC Scientific Document Group, ESC Committee for Practice Guidelines (CPG), ESC National Cardiac Societies. 2017 ESC focused update on dual antiplatelet therapy in coronary artery disease developed in collaboration with EACTS: the task force for dual antiplatelet therapy in coronary artery disease of the European Society of Cardiology (ESC) and of the European Association for Cardio-Thoracic Surgery (EACTS). Eur Heart J 2018;39:213–60.

2. Levine GN, Bates ER, Bittl JA, et al. 2016 ACC/AHA guideline focused update on duration of dual antiplatelet therapy in patients with coronary artery disease: a report of the American College of Cardiology/American Heart Association task force on clinical practice guidelines. J Am Coll Cardiol 2016;68:1082–115.

3. Franchi F, Angiolillo DJ. Novel antiplatelet agents in acute coronary syndrome. Nat Rev Cardiol 2015;12:30–47.

4. Capranzano P, Capodanno D. Switching between P2Y12 inhibitors: rationale, methods, and expected consequences. Vascul Pharmacol 2019;116:4–7.

5. Rollini F, Franchi F, Angiolillo DJ. Switching P2Y12 receptor inhibiting therapies. Interv Cardiol Clin 2017;6:67–89.

6. Rollini F, Franchi F, Angiolillo DJ. Switching P2Y12-receptor inhibitors in patients with coronary artery disease. Nat Rev Cardiol 2016;13:11–27.

7. Farid NA, Kurihara A, Wrighton SA. Metabolism and disposition of the thienopyridine antiplatelet drugs ticlopidine, clopidogrel, and prasugrel in humans. J Clin Pharmacol 2010;50:126–42.

8. Capranzano P, Ferreiro JL, Angiolillo DJ. Prasugrel in acute coronary syndrome patients undergoing percutaneous coronary intervention. Expert Rev Cardiovasc Ther 2009;7:361–9.

9. Price MJ, Walder JS, Baker BA, et al. Recovery of platelet function after discontinuation of prasugrel or clopidogrel maintenance dosing in aspirin-treated patients with stable coronary disease: the recovery trial. J Am Coll Cardiol 2012;59:2338–43.

10. Capodanno D, Dharmashankar K, Angiolillo DJ. Mechanism of action and clinical development of ticagrelor, a novel platelet ADP P2Y12 receptor antagonist. Expert Rev Cardiovasc Ther 2010;8: 151–8.

11. Gurbel PA, Bliden KP, Butler K, et al. Randomized double-blind assessment of the ONSET and OFFSET of the antiplatelet effects of ticagrelor versus clopidogrel in patients with stable coronary artery disease: the ONSET/OFFSET study. Circulation 2009;120:2577–85.

12. Angiolillo DJ, Capranzano P. Pharmacology of emerging novel platelet inhibitors. Am Heart J 2008;156:S10–5.

13. Rollini F, Franchi F, Thano E, et al. In vitro pharmacodynamic effects of cangrelor on platelet P2Y12 receptor-mediated signaling in ticagrelor-treated patients. JACC Cardiovasc Interv 2017; 10:1374–5.

14. Rollini F, Franchi F, Tello-Montoliu A, et al. Pharmacodynamic effects of cangrelor on platelet P2Y12 receptor-mediated signaling in prasugrel-treated patients. JACC Cardiovasc Interv 2014;7:426–34.

15. Angiolillo DJ, Rollini F, Storey RF, et al. International expert consensus on switching platelet P2Y12 receptor-inhibiting therapies. Circulation 2017;136:1955–75.

16. Alexopoulos D, Xanthopoulou I, Gkizas V, et al. Randomized assessment of ticagrelor versus prasugrel antiplatelet effects in patients with ST-segment-elevation myocardial infarction. Circ Cardiovasc Interv 2012;5:797e804.

17. Capodanno D, Alfonso F, Levine GN, et al. ACC/AHA versus ESC guidelines on dual antiplatelet therapy: JACC guideline comparison. J Am Coll Cardiol 2018;72:2915–31.

18. Wiviott SD, Trenk D, Frelinger AL, et al, PRINCIPLE-TIMI 44 Investigators. Prasugrel compared with high loading- and maintenance-dose clopidogrel in patients with planned percutaneous coronary intervention: the prasugrel in comparison to clopidogrel for inhibition of platelet activation and aggregation-thrombolysis in myocardial Infarction 44 trial. Circulation 2007;116:2923–32.

19. Montalescot G, Sideris G, Cohen R, et al. Prasugrel compared with high-dose clopidogrel in acute coronary syndrome. The randomised, double-blind ACAPULCO study. Thromb Haemost 2010;103: 213–23.

20. Sardella G, Calcagno S, Mancone M, et al. Pharmacodynamic effect of switching therapy in patients with high on-treatment platelet reactivity and genotype variation with high clopidogrel Dose versus prasugrel: the RESET GENE trial. Circ Cardiovasc Interv 2012;5:698–704.

21. Gurbel P, Bliden KP, Butler K, et al. Response to ticagrelor in clopidogrel nonresponders and responders and effect of switching therapies: the RESPOND study. Circulation 2010;121:1188–99.

22. Trenk D, Stone GW, Gawaz M, et al. A randomized trial of prasugrel versus clopidogrel in patients with high platelet reactivity on clopidogrel after elective percutaneous coronary intervention with implantation of drug-eluting stents: results of the TRIGGER-PCI (Testing Platelet Reactivity In Patients Undergoing Elective Stent Placement on Clopidogrel to Guide Alternative Therapy With Prasugrel) study. J Am Coll Cardiol 2012;59:2159–64.

23. Cuisset T, Gaborit B, Dubois N, et al. Platelet reactivity in diabetic patients undergoing coronary stenting for acute coronary syndrome treated with clopidogrel loading dose followed by prasugrel maintenance therapy. Int J Cardiol 2013;168:523–8.

24. Aradi D, Tornyos A, Pinter T, et al. Optimizing P2Y12 receptor inhibition in patients with acute coronary syndrome on the basis of platelet function testing: impact of prasugrel and high- dose clopidogrel. J Am Coll Cardiol 2014;63:1061–70.

25. Mayer K, Schulz S, Bernlochner I, et al. A comparative cohort study on personalised antiplatelet therapy in PCI-treated patients with high on-clopidogrel platelet reactivity. Results of the ISAR-HPR registry. Thromb Haemost 2014;112:342–51.

26. Capranzano P, Tamburino C, Capodanno D, et al. Platelet function profiles in the elderly: results of a pharmacodynamic study in patients on clopidogrel therapy and effects of switching to prasugrel 5 mg in patients with high platelet reactivity. Thromb Haemost 2011;106:1149–57.

27. Rollini F, Franchi F, Cho JR, et al. A head-to-head pharmacodynamic comparison of prasugrel vs. ticagrelor after switching from clopidogrel in patients with coronary artery disease: results of a prospective randomized study. Eur Heart J 2016;37:2722–30.

28. Alexopoulos D, Galati A, Xanthopoulou I, et al. Ticagrelor versus prasugrel in acute coronary syndrome patients with high on-clopidogrel platelet reactivity following percutaneous coronary intervention: a pharmacodynamic study. J Am Coll Cardiol 2012;60:193–9.

29. Diodati JG, Saucedo JF, French JK, et al. Effect on platelet reactivity from a prasugrel loading dose after a clopidogrel loading dose compared with a prasugrel loading dose alone: transferring from clopidogrel loading dose to prasugrel loading dose in acute coronary syndrome patients (TRIPLET): a randomized controlled trial. Circ Cardiovasc Interv 2013;6:567–74.

30. Koul S, Andell P, Martinsson A, et al. A pharmacodynamic comparison of 5 anti-platelet protocols in patients with ST-elevation myocardial infarction undergoing primary PCI. BMC Cardiovasc Disord 2014;14:189.

31. Nührenberg TG, Trenk D, Leggewie S, et al. Clopidogrel pretreatment of patients with ST-elevation myocardial infarction does not affect platelet reactivity after subsequent prasugrel-loading: platelet reactivity in an observational study. Platelets 2013;24:549–53.

32. Parodi G, De Luca G, Bellandi B, et al. Switching from clopidogrel to prasugrel in patients having coronary stent implantation. J Thromb Thrombolysis 2014;38:395–401.

33. Lhermusier T, Lipinski MJ, Drenning D, et al. Switching patients from clopidogrel to prasugrel in acute coronary syndrome: impact of the clopidogrel loading dose on platelet reactivity. J Interv Cardiol 2014;27:365–72.

34. Hibbert B, Maze R, Pourdjabbar A, et al. A comparative pharmacodynamic study of ticagrelor versus clopidogrel and ticagrelor in patients undergoing primary percutaneous coronary intervention: the CAPITAL RELOAD study. PLoS One 2014;9:e92078.

35. Payne CD, Li YG, Brandt JT, et al. Switching directly to prasugrel from clopidogrel results in greater inhibition of platelet aggregation in aspirin-treated subjects. Platelets 2008;19:275–81.

36. Angiolillo DJ, Saucedo JF, Deraad R, et al, SWAP Investigators. Increased platelet inhibition after switching from maintenance clopidogrel to prasugrel in patients with acute coronary syndromes: results of the SWAP (SWitching Anti Platelet) study. J Am Coll Cardiol 2010;56:1017–23.

37. Lhermusier T, Voisin S, Murat G, et al. Switching patients from clopidogrel to novel P2Y12 receptor inhibitors in acute coronary syndrome: comparative effects of prasugrel and ticagrelor on platelet reactivity. Int J Cardiol 2014;174:874–6.

38. Caiazzo G, De Rosa S, Torella D, et al. Administration of a loading dose has no additive effect on platelet aggregation during the switch from ongoing clopidogrel treatment to ticagrelor in patients with acute coronary syndrome. Circ Cardiovasc Interv 2014;7:104–12.

39. Wiviott SD, Braunwald E, McCabe CH, et al, TRITON-TIMI 38 Investigators. Prasugrel versus clopidogrel in patients with acute coronary syndromes. N Engl J Med 2007;357:2001–15.

40. Wallentin L, Becker RC, Budaj A, et al, PLATO Investigators. Ticagrelor versus clopidogrel in patients with acute coronary syndromes. N Engl J Med 2009;36:1045–57.

41. Clemmensen P, Grieco N, Ince H, et al, MULTIPRAC study investigators. MULTInational non-

interventional study of patients with ST-segment elevation myocardial infarction treated with PRimary Angioplasty and Concomitant use of upstream antiplatelet therapy with prasugrel or clopidogrel: the European MULTIPRAC Registry. Eur Heart J Acute Cardiovasc Care 2015;4:220–9.

42. Bagai A, Peterson ED, Honeycutt E, et al. In-hospital switching between adenosine diphosphate receptor inhibitors in patients with acute myocardial infarction treated with percutaneous coronary intervention: insights into contemporary practice from the TRANSLATEACS study. Eur Heart J Acute Cardiovasc Care 2015;4:499–508.

43. Kerneis M, Silvain J, Abtan J, et al. Switching acute coronary syndrome patients from prasugrel to clopidogrel. JACC Cardiovasc Interv 2013;6:158–65.

44. Deharo P, Pons C, Pankert M, et al. Effectiveness of switching 'hyper responders' from Prasugrel to Clopidogrel after acute coronary syndrome: the POBA (Predictor of Bleeding with Antiplatelet drugs) SWITCH study. Int J Cardiol 2013;168:5004–5.

45. Pourdjabbar A, Hibbert B, Chong AY, et al, CAPITAL Investigators. A randomised study for optimising crossover from ticagrelor to clopidogrel in patients with acute coronary syndrome. The CAPITAL OPTI-CROSS Study. Thromb Haemost 2017;117:303–10.

46. Franchi F, Rollini F, Rivas Rios J, et al. Pharmacodynamic effects of switching from ticagrelor to clopidogrel in patients with coronary artery disease: results of the SWAP-4 study. Circulation 2018;137:2450–62.

47. Antman EM, Wiviott SD, Murphy SA, et al. Early and late benefits of prasugrel in patients with acute coronary syndromes undergoing percutaneous coronary intervention: a TRITON-TIMI 38 (TRial to Assess Improvement in Therapeutic Outcomes by Optimizing Platelet InhibitioN with Prasugrel-Thrombolysis In Myocardial Infarction) analysis. J Am Coll Cardiol 2008;51:2028–33.

48. Becker RC, Bassand JP, Budaj A, et al. Bleeding complications with the P2Y12 receptor antagonists clopidogrel and ticagrelor in the PLATelet inhibition and patient Outcomes (PLATO) trial. Eur Heart J 2011;32:2933–44.

49. Cuisset T, Deharo P, Quillici J, et al. Benefit of switching dual antiplatelet therapy after acute coronary syndrome: the TOPIC (timing of platelet inhibition after acute coronary syndrome) randomized study. Eur Heart J 2017;38:3070–8.

50. Sibbing D, Aradi D, Jacobshagen C, et al. Guided de-escalation of antiplatelet treatment in patients with acute coronary syndrome undergoing percutaneous coronary intervention (TROPICAL-ACS): a randomized, open-label, multicenter trial. Lancet 2017;390:1747–57.

51. Deharo P, Quilici J, Camoin-Jau L, et al. Benefit of switching dual antiplatelet therapy after acute coronary syndrome according to on-treatment platelet reactivity: the TOPIC-VASP pre-specified analysis of the TOPIC randomized study. JACC Cardiovasc Interv 2017;10:2560–70.

52. Aradi D, Gross L, Trenk, et al. Platelet reactivity and clinical outcomes in acute coronary syndrome patients treated with prasugrel and clopidogrel: a pre-specified exploratory analysis from the TROPICAL-ACS trial. Eur Heart J 2019;40:1942–51.

53. Neumann FJ, Sousa-Uva M, Ahlsson A, et al. 2018 ESC/EACTS guidelines on myocardial revascularization. Eur Heart J 2019;40:87–165.

54. Moon JY, Franchi F, Rollini F, et al. Role of genetic testing in patients undergoing percutaneous coronary intervention. Expert Rev Clin Pharmacol 2018;11:151–64.

55. Sibbing D, Aradi D, Alexopoulos D, et al. Updated expert consensus statement on platelet function and genetic testing for guiding P2Y$_{12}$ receptor inhibitor treatment in percutaneous coronary intervention. JACC Cardiovasc Interv 2019. [Epub ahead of print].

56. Angiolillo DJ, Curzen N, Gurbel P, et al. Pharmacodynamic evaluation of switching from ticagrelor to prasugrel in patients with stable coronary artery disease: results of the SWAP-2 Study (Switching Anti Platelet-2). J Am Coll Cardiol 2014;63:1500–9.

57. Franchi F, Faz GT, Rollini F, et al. Pharmacodynamic effects of switching from prasugrel to ticagrelor: results of the prospective, randomized SWAP-3 study. JACC Cardiovasc Interv 2016;9:1089–98.

58. Bhatt DL, Stone GW, Mahaffey KW, et al, CHAMPION PHOENIX Investigators. Effect of platelet inhibition with cangrelor during PCI on ischemic events. N Engl J Med 2013;368:1303–13.

59. Steinhubl SR, Oh JJ, Oestreich JH, et al. Transitioning patients from cangrelor to clopidogrel: pharmacodynamic evidence of a competitive effect. Thromb Res 2008;121:527–34.

60. Schneider DJ, Agarwal Z, Seecheran N, et al. Pharmacodynamic effects when clopidogrel is given before cangrelor discontinuation. J Interv Cardiol 2015;28:415–9.

61. Angiolillo DJ, Schneider DJ, Bhatt DL, et al. Pharmacodynamic effects of cangrelor and clopidogrel: the platelet function substudy from the cangrelor versus standard therapy to achieve optimal management of platelet inhibition (CHAMPION) trials. J Thromb Thrombolysis 2012;34:44–55.

62. Schneider DJ, Agarwal Z, Seecheran N, et al. Pharmacodynamic effects during the transition between cangrelor and ticagrelor. JACC Cardiovasc Interv 2014;7:435–42.

63. Schneider DJ, Seecheran N, Raza SS, et al. Pharmacodynamic effects during the transition between

cangrelor and prasugrel. Coron Artery Dis 2015;26:
42–8.

64. Hochholzer W, Kleiner P, Younas I, et al. Randomized comparison of oral P2Y12-receptor inhibitor
loading strategies for transitioning from cangrelor:
the ExcelsiorLOAD2 trial. JACC Cardiovasc Interv
2017;10:121–9.

65. Franchi F, Rollini F, Rivas A, et al. Platelet inhibition
with cangrelor and crushed ticagrelor in patients
with ST-elevation myocardial infarction undergoing
primary percutaneous coronary intervention: results
of the CANTIC study. Circulation 2019;139:1661–70.

66. Capranzano P, Capodanno D, Bucciarelli-Ducci C,
et al. Impact of residual platelet reactivity on

reperfusion in patients with ST-segment elevation
myocardial infarction undergoing primary percutaneous coronary intervention. Eur Heart J Acute Cardiovasc Care 2016;5:475–86.

67. Angiolillo DJ, Firstenberg MS, Price MJ, et al,
BRIDGE Investigators. Bridging antiplatelet therapy with cangrelor in patients undergoing cardiac
surgery: a randomized controlled trial. JAMA
2012;307:265–74.

68. Rossini R, Tarantini G, Musumeci G, et al.
A multidisciplinary approach on the perioperative
antithrombotic management of patients with coronary stents undergoing surgery: surgery after stenting 2. JACC Cardiovasc Interv 2018;11:417–34.

Transcatheter Closure of Patent Foramen Ovale
Randomized Trial Update

Angelos Arfaras-Melainis, MD[a,1],
Leonidas Palaiodimos, MD, MSc[b,*],
Mohammad K. Mojadidi, MD[c,2]

KEYWORDS

- PFO • Cryptogenic stroke • PFO closure • Embolic stroke of undetermined source • ESUS
- Stroke prevention

KEY POINTS

- Recent randomized trials have proven the superiority of percutaneous patent foramen ovale (PFO) closure over standard-of-care antithrombotic agents for patients ≤60 years old with stroke of unknown cause other than PFO.
- Ischemic stroke patients who have PFO with high-risk features (ie, atrial septal aneurysm, substantial shunt through a large PFO, Eustachian valve, or Chiari network) appeared to benefit the most from device closure. Experts consider a high-risk PFO to be an enhanced reason for percutaneous closure.
- Although PFO closure is associated with a 4-fold increased risk of new-onset atrial fibrillation in the periprocedural period, the stroke risk linked to this type of atrial fibrillation appears to be minimal (~0.1%).
- Percutaneous PFO closure is a safe procedure associated with very low risk of complications; in the cardiology community, it is often considered the safest therapeutic interventional cardiology procedure.
- Further studies are needed to evaluate the efficacy and safety of percutaneous PFO closure in elderly patients with PFO-mediated stroke, the role of this procedure for primary prevention in patients with high-risk PFO, and the optimal duration of postprocedural antiplatelet therapy.

INTRODUCTION

The incidence of ischemic stroke in the United States approaches 800,000 cases per year.[1] Of these, a clear cause cannot be identified in 20% to 30% after the initial standard workup; these strokes are subsequently termed, "cryptogenic."[1] A patent foramen ovale (PFO) is a congenital cardiac defect of the atrial septum and remnant of the fetal circulation that can function as a transient, interatrial right-to-left shunt. It is common and present in one-quarter of all adults; in comparison, 40% to 60% of patients with otherwise cryptogenic

Conflict of Interest Disclosure: No conflict of interest.
Funding: No funding was available for this study.
[a] Second Cardiology Department, National and Kapodistrian University of Athens, Attikon University Hospital, 1 Rimini Street, Haidari, Athens 12462, Greece; [b] Department of Medicine, Division of Hospital Medicine, Montefiore Medical Center, Albert Einstein College of Medicine, 111 East 210th Street, Bronx, NY 10467, USA; [c] Division of Cardiology, Department of Medicine, Virginia Commonwealth University, 1101 East Marshall Street, Richmond, VA 23298, USA
[1] Present address: 19 Kleisouras Street, Attica, Athens 14542, Greece.
[2] Present address: 1755 North Mecklenburg Avenue, South Hill, VA 23950.
* Corresponding author.
E-mail address: leonidas.palaiodimos@gmail.com

Intervent Cardiol Clin 8 (2019) 341–356
https://doi.org/10.1016/j.iccl.2019.05.002
2211-7458/19/© 2019 Elsevier Inc. All rights reserved.

stroke are found to have a PFO.[2–4] Since the first description of an occluded cerebral artery in a young patient with a PFO and concomitant deep vein thrombosis more than a century ago,[5] the mechanism that links PFO and stroke is paradoxical embolism. It is now widely accepted that a thrombus arising in the venous circulation can cross the interatrial septum via the PFO, resulting in arterial embolization to the brain (stroke), heart (myocardial infarction), or systemic circulation (peripheral ischemia).[6–8]

In addition, certain coexisting regional anatomic variations can open the PFO more frequently, causing interatrial right-to-left shunting and an increased risk of stroke.[9] Specifically, some patients have a localized saccular deformity of the atrial septum that is called an atrial septal aneurysm; this deformity has been associated with a 5-fold increased risk of an initial stroke and 20-fold increased risk of a recurrent event.[10,11] Other anatomic variants, such as the Eustachian valve and Chiari network, may facilitate a stroke by directing lower-body venous thrombi from the inferior vena cava straight into the PFO opening.[12,13] In addition to paradoxical embolism engendering stroke, myocardial infarction, and peripheral ischemia, a PFO has also been associated with a variety of other conditions, including migraine with aura, hypoxemia-related conditions, and decompression sickness.[14–22]

The concept of percutaneous closure of PFO for secondary prevention of paradoxic embolism-mediated stroke initially arose about 30 years ago.[23] A large meta-analysis of 48 early observational studies found that in patients with otherwise cryptogenic stroke or transient ischemic attack (TIA), percutaneous PFO device closure reduced the risk of recurrent neurologic events by 6.3-fold when compared with standard-of-care medical therapy.[24] Subsequently, 6 randomized controlled trials were completed, which compared the efficacy and safety of percutaneous PFO closure versus medical therapy for secondary prevention stroke. This review summarizes the randomized trials of PFO closure for stroke, with an emphasis on the lessons learned from these studies, and how the data can be applied to everyday clinical practice to treat stroke patients who are found to have PFO on echocardiography.

DIAGNOSIS AND QUANTIFICATION OF PATENT FORAMEN OVALE

The most accurate method to confirm a PFO is a right heart catheterization, whereby the PFO can be documented with passing of a guidewire through the interatrial septum under fluoroscopy, or with angiographic injection of radiopaque contrast into the PFO to visualize the right-to-left shunt (a so-called right atriogram).[25,26] However, the interventional nature of this technique limits its use as an initial screening modality.[27]

Transesophageal echocardiography (TEE) with agitated saline bubble study is considered the minimally invasive reference standard for the detection and quantification of PFO-mediated right-to-left shunting. It allows a detailed assessment of the PFO anatomy, diagnosis of coexisting anatomic variants, and differentiation between a PFO, atrial septal defect, and pulmonary shunt.[22,23] However, a TEE is found to either miss or misdiagnose a PFO in about 10% of cases when compared with confirmation during cardiac catheterization, autopsy, and/or surgery as the reference.[28] In addition, the invasive nature of TEE may pose some limitations, such as patient discomfort (including swallowing difficulty that is common in stroke patients) and the need for sedation.[27] Therefore, other imaging modalities, such as transthoracic echocardiography (TTE) and transcranial Doppler (TCD), both with agitated saline bubble study, are commonly used as initial screening tests. TCD offers a higher sensitivity but lower specificity (sensitivity of 97% and specificity of 93%) when compared with TEE as the reference[27]; it has the advantage of accurately quantifying a residual shunt after PFO closure,[27,29] but has the disadvantage of not being able to differentiate between a PFO, atrial septal defect, and pulmonary shunt.[30] TTE with fundamental imaging is the least sensitive modality, with a sensitivity of only 46%,[30] which, however, reaches up to 90% when performed on harmonic imaging mode.[31–33] All of these studies of different imaging modalities are flawed, however, because they used TEE as the reference standard rather than cardiac catheterization; only a right heart catheterization can most accurately document or exclude a PFO (Table 1).

PATENT FORAMEN OVALE AND STROKE: EARLY RANDOMIZED TRIALS

Before completion of the initial trials of PFO closure for stroke, observational data had already demonstrated that approximately half of patients with otherwise cryptogenic stroke have a PFO.[2–4] This observation suggested that PFO-mediated paradoxical embolism could be

Table 1
Imaging modalities for the diagnosis of patent foramen ovale and their associated characteristics

Modality	Sensitivity, %	Specificity, %	Advantages	Disadvantages
TEE[a]	90	>95	PFO vs ASD or pulmonary shunt, direct visualization	Patient discomfort, sedation
TCD[b]	97	93	Highest sensitivity, postprocedural residual shunt quantification	Unable to differentiate cardiac vs intrapulmonary shunt
TTE[b]	50–60 90 (with harmonic imaging)	>90	Excellent specificity, widely available	Poor sensitivity without harmonic imaging

Abbreviation: ASD, atrial septal defect.
[a] Compared with right-heart catheterization, surgery, or autopsy.
[b] Compared with TEE.

the underlying pathophysiology for many of these strokes. Results of the Clinical and Imaging Findings in Cryptogenic Stroke Patients with and without Patent Foramen Ovale (PFO-ASA) study reinforced this hypothesis.[34] PFO-ASA was a multicenter prospective study investigating risk factors and patterns in patients with and without PFO and cryptogenic stroke. The results showed that patients with a PFO were significantly different from patients without PFO in terms of age (40.1 years vs 44.5 years, P<.001) and cardiovascular risk factors (eg, hypertension, 8.6% vs 21.3%, P<.001).[34]

Numerous observational studies and their meta-analyses demonstrated that PFO closure appeared to prevent recurrent stroke in these young and otherwise healthy patients with stroke of no other identifiable cause. Between 2012 and 2013, 3 randomized trials assessed the efficacy and safety of percutaneous device closure compared with standard-of-care medical therapy for secondary prevention of ischemic stroke from no other apparent cause other than PFO[35–37] (Table 2).

CLOSURE I Trial

The Evaluation of the STARFlex Septal Closure System in Patients with a Stroke and/or Transient Ischemic Attack due to Presumed Paradoxical Embolism through a PFO (CLOSURE I) trial was the first randomized, multicenter, open-label study of the safety and efficacy of PFO closure. It enrolled 909 patients, all of whom were 60 years of age or younger.[32] The follow-up period was 2 years. The scope of the trial was to assess the utility of percutaneous PFO closure plus medical treatment versus medical therapy alone in patients with otherwise cryptogenic stroke or TIA. The presence of PFO was confirmed by TEE. Patients were randomly

assigned to device closure with the STARFlex septal closure system (NMT Medical, Boston, MA, USA) plus antiplatelets (aspirin for 2 years and clopidogrel for 6 months) or to antithrombotic treatment only (warfarin, aspirin, or both). The primary endpoint was a composite of recurrent stroke or TIA in 2 years, death from any cause during the first 30 days, or death from neurologic causes between 31 days and 2 years. The primary endpoint was met in 5.5% (23 of 447) of patients in the device group and in 6.8% (29 of 462) of patients in the medical therapy group (hazard ratio [HR] 0.78, 95% confidence interval [CI] 0.45–1.35, P = .37). PFO closure did not appear to significantly decrease the rate of recurrent stroke when compared with medical therapy (2.9% vs 3.1%, P = .79) or TIA (3.1% vs 4.1%, P = .44).

It is noteworthy that PFO closure with the STARFlex device was associated with an increased risk of major vascular complications (3.2% vs 0%, P<.001) and new-onset atrial fibrillation (5.7% vs 0.7%, P<.001), which raised significant safety concerns. Specifically, 26 patients developed new-onset atrial fibrillation (23 of them in the device group), of whom 3 had recurrent stroke during the follow-up period, presumably from device-associated atrial fibrillation. In addition, during a 6-month follow-up, 14% of patients with a device had significant residual right-to-left shunting on echocardiography. Moreover, 4 patients in the device group (1.1%) had a new atrial thrombus identified during the same visit, and 2 out of these 4 patients had recurrent stroke. Adding to data from earlier observational studies, the safety results from CLOSURE I led to the conjecture that the STARFlex device is associated with increased risk of thrombus formation, atrial fibrillation, and considerable

Table 2
Early randomized controlled trials of patent foramen ovale closure for secondary stroke prevention

Study	Number of Patients	Inclusion Criteria	Device	Follow-up, y	Antithrombotic Therapy	Primary Endpoint	Result
CLOSURE I	909	Patients 16–60 y old & cryptogenic stroke or TIA & PFO	STARFlex septal closure system	2	Device arm: Aspirin & warfarin (1 mo) followed by aspirin (2 y) Medical treatment arm: Aspirin or warfarin or aspirin & warfarin	Early all-cause death, late death due to neurologic cause, stroke, TIA	Percutaneous PFO closure did not significantly reduce recurrent stroke or TIA compared with medical treatment alone
PC	414	Patients <60 y old with cryptogenic stroke, TIA, or systemic embolism & PFO	Amplatzer PFO Occluder	4	Device arm: Aspirin (5–6 mo) & ticlopidine or clopidogrel (1–6 mo) Medical treatment arm: Antiplatelet therapy or anticoagulation therapy	Death, nonfatal stroke, TIA, or peripheral embolism	Percutaneous PFO closure did not significantly reduce death or recurrent embolism compared with medical treatment alone
RESPECT	980	Patients 18–60 y old & cryptogenic stroke & PFO	Amplatzer PFO Occluder	5.9 (median)	Device arm: Aspirin plus clopidogrel (1 mo), followed by aspirin (5 mo) Medical treatment arm: Aspirin or warfarin or clopidogrel or aspirin and extended-release dipyridamole	Recurrent fatal and nonfatal stroke and early death	Percutaneous PFO closure significantly reduced recurrent stroke rates compared with medical treatment alone

residual shunting.[36,38–40] This device is no longer manufactured.

The PC Trial

The Percutaneous Closure of Patent Foramen Ovale in Cryptogenic Embolism (PC) trial was published in 2013, 1 year after the CLOSURE I trial.[37] The study enrolled 414 patients younger than 60 years of age, with a TEE-confirmed PFO and a recent history of ischemic stroke, TIA with abnormal cerebral imaging, or a peripheral thromboembolic event. The follow-up period of this study was 4 years. Individuals were randomized to PFO closure with the Amplatzer PFO Occluder (Abbott Vascular, Minneapolis, MN, USA) plus aspirin and clopidogrel or ticlopidine, or to standard-of-care medical treatment with antiplatelets or anticoagulants, selected at the discretion of the treating neurologist. The primary endpoint, a composite of death, nonfatal stroke, TIA, or peripheral embolism, occurred in 3.4% (7/204) of patients in the device arm and in 5.2% (11/210) of patients in the medical therapy arm (HR 0.63, 95% CI 0.24–1.62, $P = .34$). The incidence of serious adverse events in the 2 study arms did not significantly differ, including new-onset atrial fibrillation (6 cases in device group vs 2 cases in medical therapy group, $P = .17$) and major bleeding (1 case in device group vs 3 cases in medical therapy group, $P = .62$).

The PC trial was statistically underpowered to detect differences in clinical events between the 2 treatment strategies. In addition, this trial enrolled not only patients with a cerebrovascular event but also patients with peripheral embolism, a cohort that was different from the traditional stroke patients included in the observational studies.

The RESPECT Trial

The early results of the Randomized Evaluation of Recurrent Stroke Comparing PFO Closure to Established Current Standard of Care Treatment (RESPECT) trial were published in 2013.[35] A cohort of 980 stroke patients, 60 years of age or younger, were assigned to transcatheter PFO closure with the Amplatzer PFO Occluder or standard-of-care medical therapy. The choice of medical therapy included 4 different regimens (aspirin, warfarin, clopidogrel, or aspirin plus dipyridamole) that were left at the discretion of the treating neurologist. The primary endpoint was a composite of recurrent nonfatal ischemic stroke, fatal ischemic stroke, or early death. A key difference in the design of this study, compared with CLOSURE I and PC, is that the

RESPECT trial did not have a prespecified follow-up period, but was designed to continue until a target of 25 primary endpoint events were observed. This event-driven follow-up design of the RESPECT trial led to an early follow-up phase that was completed when 25 occurrences occurred (median follow-up, 2.1 years), and a late follow-up phase until a regulatory decision was made, thus accumulating a total of 5688 efficacy and 5810 safety patient-years of follow-up (median follow-up, 5.9 years).

Although the early RESPECT data (median follow-up 2.1 years) could not statistically demonstrate superiority of PFO closure over medical therapy for secondary stroke prevention in the intention-to-treat analysis (0.7% vs 1.4%; HR 0.49, 95% CI 0.22–1.11, $P = .08$),[35] the long-term follow-up data (median follow-up 5.9 years) showed a significant reduction in recurrent stroke in the device arm when compared with medical therapy (3.6% vs 5.8%, HR 0.55%, 95% CI 0.31–0.999, $P = .046$).[41] The results remained significant despite the fact that 3 patients who were randomized to the device arm did not actually receive a device, but had recurrent stroke. The benefit of PFO closure appeared to be more prominent in subgroups of patients with coexisting anatomic variations, notably those with a large shunt (2.0% vs 6.9%; HR 0.26, 95% CI 0.10–0.71, $P = .005$, interaction $P = .04$) or atrial septal aneurysm (1.7% vs 7.6%; HR 0.20, 95% CI 0.06–0.70, $P = .005$, interaction $P = .04$). With respect to safety, there were no significant differences in adjudicated serious adverse events between the 2 study arms, and the rate of atrial fibrillation after the periprocedural period did not differ significantly (HR 1.47, 95% CI 0.64–3.37, $P = .36$).

One important limitation of the RESPECT trial was the different rates of patient dropout between the 2 groups, especially in the long-term phase of the study. The percentage of patients who dropped out of the device arm was 20.8%, whereas it was 33.3% in the medical treatment arm. A higher dropout rate in the medical therapy group may have altered the duration of meaningful follow-up for possible stroke recurrence between the 2 groups.

Meta-Analyses of the Early Three Trials

Following publication of the early trials of PFO closure for stroke (CLOSURE I, PC, and early RESPECT), several meta-analyses were conducted with the goal to increase statistical power and decrease risk of type II error, a potential limitation of all the studies.[42–44] A patient level meta-analysis by Kent and colleagues[44] pooled the individual data of 2303 patients from the 3 trials; the collective analysis showed that PFO closure was superior to medical therapy for secondary prevention of stroke (HR 0.58; 95% CI 0.34–0.98, P = .043). There was an enhanced clinical yield in the subgroup analysis for patients who received the Amplatzer PFO Occluder (HR 0.39; 95% CI 0.19–0.82, P = .013).[44] The findings of this meta-analysis, along with the long-term data of the RESPECT trial, led to the premarket approval of the Amplatzer PFO Occluder by the Food and Drug Administration (FDA) in October 2016 for use in patients, 18 to 60 years of age, with stroke determined by a neurologist and cardiologist to be due to paradoxical embolism.[45]

PATENT FORAMEN OVALE AND STROKE: RECENT RANDOMIZED CONTROLLED TRIALS

More recently, 3 international randomized trials evaluated the efficacy and safety of PFO device closure over standard-of-care medical therapy in patients with ischemic stroke of no other apparent cause other than PFO. These new studies have expanded the understanding of PFO-mediated stroke and allowed us to identify which stroke patients would benefit most from percutaneous device closure[46–48] (Table 3).

The Gore REDUCE Trial

The Gore Helex Septal Occluder/Gore Cardioform Septal Occluder and Antiplatelet Medical Management for Reduction of Recurrent Stroke or Imaging-Confirmed Transient Ischemic Attack in Patients with PFO (REDUCE) trial was published in 2017.[46] The study included 664 patients younger than 60 years of age, with a recent diagnosis of ischemic stroke and no other identifiable culprits other than a TEE-confirmed PFO. Patients were randomly assigned in a 2:1 ratio to PFO closure plus antiplatelet therapy versus antiplatelets alone and followed for a median of 3.2 years. Those who underwent PFO closure had significantly lower rates of stroke recurrence both clinically (1.4% vs 5.4%; HR 0.23; 95% CI 0.09–0.62; P = .002) and radiographically (5.7% vs 11.3%; risk ratio 0.51; 95% CI 0.29–0.91; P = .04). The number needed to treat (NNT) to prevent 1 stroke in 24 months was calculated to be as low as 28. The incidence of serious adverse events, including major bleeding and venous thromboembolism, was similar between the 2 groups. However, there was a significantly higher rate of atrial fibrillation or flutter documented in the closure group when compared

with medical therapy (6.6% vs 0.4%, P<.001). Similar to the results of the CLOSE trial, most device-associated atrial arrhythmias occurred early after the procedure (first 45 days), most of which (59%) resolved within 2 weeks. Even though the rate of overall atrial fibrillation was higher in the device arm, the rate of atrial fibrillation adjudicated because a serious adverse did not differ significantly between the 2 arms. The difference in dropout rates between the 2 groups (8.8% in device arm vs 14.8% in medical therapy arm) may have affected the overall analysis and interpretation of the results.

The Gore REDUCE trial was in agreement with the extended follow-up results of the RESPECT trial, showing that all young patients with stroke attributed to PFO will have less recurrent stroke events compared with standard-of-care medical therapy on long-term follow-up, with no difference in serious adverse events or influence on major bleeding.

The CLOSE Trial

The Patent Foramen Ovale Closure or Anticoagulants versus Antiplatelet Therapy to Prevent Stroke Recurrence (CLOSE) trial was published in 2017.[47] The study enrolled 663 patients aged 60 years or younger, with a history of recent stroke of no other identifiable cause other than PFO. In an effort to only include stroke that is more likely attributable to paradoxical embolism, the trial only enrolled patients with high-risk anatomic features by echocardiography (ie, presence of atrial septal aneurysm or substantial shunt). Subjects were randomized into 1 of 3 arms. The first group received percutaneous PFO closure with 1 of 11 different closure devices plus antiplatelet therapy; the second group was treated with antiplatelet therapy alone, and the third group was treated with oral anticoagulation. At a mean follow-up of 5.3 years, no recurrent stroke events were observed in the device arm, and the PFO closure group showed a markedly lower rate of recurrent stroke (in fact, 0 strokes) compared with the medical therapy group (0% vs 6.0%; HR 0.03; 95% CI 0–0.26; P<.001). The NNT to prevent 1 stroke in 5 years was 20. There was no significant difference in serious adverse events between the 3 groups (including major bleeding, death, or all-cause serious adverse events). However, the incidence of atrial fibrillation or flutter was higher in the PFO closure group (4.6% vs 0.9%; P = .02). A total of 11 cases of atrial fibrillation was documented; 91% of them occurred within the first postprocedural month and 70% did not require long-term anticoagulation. Although the rate of

Table 3
Recent randomized controlled trials of patent foramen ovale closure for secondary stroke prevention

Study	Number of Patients	Inclusion Criteria	Device	Follow-up, y	Antithrombotic Therapy	Primary Endpoint	Result
CLOSE	663	Patients 16–60 y old & cryptogenic stroke & PFO associated with an atrial septal aneurysm or large interatrial shunt	Amplatzer, STARFlex, CardioSEAL, Intrasept, PFO-Star, HELEX, Premere, Occlutech, Cardioform	5.3 (mean)	Device arm: Aspirin & clopidogrel (3 mo), followed by single antiplatelet therapy Medical treatment arm: Aspirin or clopidogrel or aspirin combined with extended-release dipyridamole or warfarin or NOAC	Recurrent stroke	Percutaneous PFO closure significantly reduces recurrent strokes compared with medical treatment alone
Gore REDUCE	664	Patients 18–59 y old & cryptogenic stroke & PFO	Helex septal occluder, Cardioform septal occluder	3.2 (median)	Device arm: Clopidogrel (first 3 d) followed by the chosen antiplatelet therapy for the medical treatment arm Medical treatment arm: Aspirin or aspirin & dipyridamole or clopidogrel	Freedom from clinical evidence of ischemic stroke and incidence of new brain infarction (clinical ischemic stroke and silent brain infarction detected on MRI)	Percutaneous PFO closure significantly reduces recurrent strokes and new brain infarcts compared with medical treatment alone
DEFENSE-PFO	120	Patients with ischemic stroke and no identifiable cause other than a high-risk PFO	Amplatzer PFO Occluder	2 (median)	Device arm: DAPT (6 mo), followed by single antiplatelet, DAPT, or anticoagulation Medical treatment arm: Aspirin, aspirin & clopidogrel, aspirin & cilostazol or warfarin	Stroke, vascular death, or TIMI-defined major bleeding	Percutaneous PFO closure significantly reduces recurrent strokes compared with medical treatment alone, in patients with high-risk PFO

Abbreviations: DAPT, dual antiplatelet therapy; NOAC, non-vitamin K oral anticoagulant; TIMI, thrombolysis in myocardial infarction.

recurrent stroke was numerically lower with oral anticoagulation compared with antiplatelet therapy, this did not reach statistical significance (1.6% vs 4.0%; HR 0.44, 95% CI 0.11–1.48); this observation was also accompanied by a numerically higher rate of bleeding with anticoagulation when compared with antiplatelet therapy (5.3% vs 2.3%; P = .18). However, it should be mentioned that this trial was not adequately powered to detect differences in events between the 2 medical therapy groups due to a lower-than-expected rate of patient recruitment and eventual early termination.

In summary, the CLOSE study, in concordance with the RESPECT trial,[41] showed that percutaneous PFO closure is superior to standard-of-care medical therapy for secondary prevention of stroke associated with PFO plus high-risk echocardiographic features.

The DEFENSE-PFO Trial

The Device Closure versus Medical Therapy for Cryptogenic Stroke Patients with High-Risk Patent Foramen Ovale (DEFENSE-PFO) trial was conducted in South Korea and published in 2018.[48] A total of 120 patients with a history of ischemic stroke of no apparent cause other than a high-risk PFO (atrial septal aneurysm, septal hypermobility, or PFO size $\geq$2 mm) was included in the study. Patients were randomized to device closure with the Amplatzer PFO Occluder or medical therapy (aspirin, aspirin plus clopidogrel, aspirin plus cilostazol, or warfarin). The primary endpoint was a composite of stroke, vascular death, or major bleeding. At a median follow-up of 2.8 years, the primary endpoint was observed in 0 patients in the device arm and 6 patients in the medical treatment arm (0% vs 12.9%, 95% CI 3.2–22.6; P = .013). PFO closure was superior to medical treatment in preventing stroke recurrence (0% vs 10.5%; 95% CI 1.68–19.32; P = .023). Regarding silent cerebral infarction, the difference was not statistically significant (8.8% vs 18.4%, P = .24). The NNT to prevent 1 stroke in 2 years was calculated as low as 10. Of note, this number may be an overestimation because of early termination of the study that led to a small cohort and decreased statistical power. The study did not show any significant periprocedural safety concerns when compared with medical therapy. Postprocedural atrial fibrillation occurred in only 2 patients in the PFO closure group.

The results of the DEFENSE-PFO study confirmed the data from the CLOSE trial, demonstrating marked superiority of percutaneous PFO closure over standard-of-care medical therapy for secondary prevention of stroke associated with high-risk PFO; both studies had substantially low NNTs when compared with the other trials.

Meta-Analyses of all Six Randomized Trials

More than a dozen meta-analyses were subsequently published to pool the data from the randomized trials, in an effort to increase the sample size and decrease risk of type II error.[49–61] All of the meta-analyses yielded a similar conclusion, showing that percutaneous PFO closure significantly decreases the risk of recurrent stroke compared with medical therapy in patients with stroke attributed to PFO; the pooled data also showed that this clinical benefit of PFO closure is accompanied by no increased risk of major adverse events or influence on major bleeding when compared with standard-of-care blood thinners (**Fig. 1**).[52] One caveat is that PFO closure was found to be associated with a 4-fold increased risk of atrial fibrillation or flutter. This difference, although present, was not as profound in the subgroup of patients who received the Amplatzer PFO Occluder (odds ratio 2.29, 95% CI 0.91–5.76).[62]

SAFETY OF PERCUTANEOUS PATENT FORAMEN OVALE CLOSURE

The randomized trials of PFO closure used several different PFO-occluding devices: the STARFlex device (no longer manufactured) was used in CLOSURE I; the Amplatzer PFO Occluder was used in PC, RESPECT, and DEFENSE-PFO; the Helex (no longer manufactured) or Cardioform septal occluders (W.L. Gore and Associates, Flagstaff, Arizona) were used in Gore REDUCE; and 1 of 11 different devices was used in the CLOSE trial.

An occasional complaint reported after device implantation is chest pain. It is hypothesized that chest pain may be a symptom of an exaggerated inflammatory response to the nickel contained in the commonly used devices.[63] In a large observational study of nearly 14,000 patients who underwent PFO closure, Verma and Tobis[63] reported that 1 in every 500 devices underwent surgical explantation, the most common reason being severe persistent chest pain likely secondary to excessive scar tissue formation due to an allergic reaction. However, the trials that reported this side effect and used the Amplatzer PFO Occluder, which has the highest nickel content, showed no significant difference in terms of chest pain between the PFO closure and the medical treatment groups.[37,41]

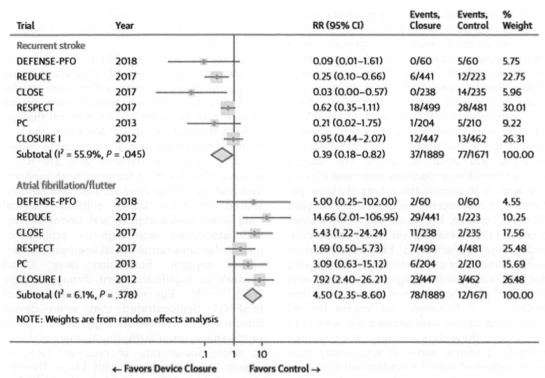

Trial	Year		RR (95% CI)	Events, Closure	Events, Control	% Weight
Recurrent stroke						
DEFENSE-PFO	2018		0.09 (0.01–1.61)	0/60	5/60	5.75
REDUCE	2017		0.25 (0.10–0.66)	6/441	12/223	22.75
CLOSE	2017		0.03 (0.00–0.57)	0/238	14/235	5.96
RESPECT	2017		0.62 (0.35–1.11)	18/499	28/481	30.01
PC	2013		0.21 (0.02–1.75)	1/204	5/210	9.22
CLOSURE I	2012		0.95 (0.44–2.07)	12/447	13/462	26.31
Subtotal (I^2 = 55.9%, P = .045)			0.39 (0.18–0.82)	37/1889	77/1671	100.00
Atrial fibrillation/flutter						
DEFENSE-PFO	2018		5.00 (0.25–102.00)	2/60	0/60	4.55
REDUCE	2017		14.66 (2.01–106.95)	29/441	1/223	10.25
CLOSE	2017		5.43 (1.22–24.24)	11/238	2/235	17.56
RESPECT	2017		1.69 (0.50–5.73)	7/499	4/481	25.48
PC	2013		3.09 (0.63–15.12)	6/204	2/210	15.69
CLOSURE I	2012		7.92 (2.40–26.21)	23/447	3/462	26.48
Subtotal (I^2 = 6.1%, P = .378)			4.50 (2.35–8.60)	78/1889	12/1671	100.00

NOTE: Weights are from random effects analysis

.1   1   10

← Favors Device Closure   Favors Control →

Fig. 1. Meta-analysis of the 6 randomized trials of PFO closure for stroke. Summary plot for primary efficacy (recurrent stroke) and primary safety (atrial fibrillation/flutter). Relative size of data markers indicates weight of sample size. RR, risk ratio. (*From* Mojadidi et al. Cryptogenic Stroke and Patent Foramen Ovale: Ready for Prime Time? J Am Coll Cardiol, 2018;72(10):1183–5. Copyright © year 2018, with permission.)

All 6 randomized trials did not demonstrate any significant difference in serious adverse events, such as major bleeding or venous thromboembolism, when PFO closure was compared with medical therapy (Table 4). It should be noted that in the RESPECT trial, the device was associated with an increased risk of pulmonary embolism (HR 3.48; 95% CI 0.98–12.34; P = .04); however, more patients had a history of venous thromboembolism events in the device arm as compared with the medical treatment arm (17/499 vs 4/481). Device-associated thrombosis only occurred in the CLOSURE I, which was reported in 2 patients; there were no reported

cases of device thrombosis in PC, RESPECT, DEFENSE-PFO, CLOSE, and REDUCE. However, the trials showed a 4-fold increased risk of new-onset atrial fibrillation or flutter in patients who received a device.[35–37,46–48,51,62]

LESSONS LEARNED AND UNANSWERED QUESTIONS

Compared with the earlier studies, the more recent randomized controlled trials implemented relatively stricter criteria for patient selection in an effort to enroll only those patients afflicted by PFO-mediated paradoxical embolism as the

Table 4
Rates of any serious adverse events and atrial fibrillation or flutter in the trials of patent foramen ovale closure for secondary stroke prevention

Study Arm	CLOSURE I Closure	MT	PC Closure	MT	RESPECT Closure	MT	CLOSE Closure	MT	Gore REDUCE Closure	MT	DEFENSE-PFO Closure	MT
Serious adverse events (%)	16.9	16.6	21.1	17.6	40.3	36	35.7	33.2	23.1	27.8	6.6	5
AF (%)	5.7	0.7	3.0	1.0	1.4	0.8	4.6	0.9	6.6	0.4	3.3	0

Abbreviation: MT, medical treatment.

likely cause of their index cerebrovascular event. Patients who were found to have intracranial or large-vessel extracranial atherosclerosis, small vessel occlusive disease (lacunar infarcts), atrial fibrillation or flutter, cardiac thrombi, hypercoagulable disorders, vasculitides, or aortic dissection were largely excluded.[46–48] Moreover, young and otherwise healthy patients aged 60 or younger were predominantly enrolled, a cohort devoid of the traditional risk factors of atherosclerosis and atrial fibrillation. The lessons learned from the randomized trials have allowed the authors to identify the cohort of stroke patients who may receive the highest clinical yield from PFO closure. The results of the randomized trials and their meta-analyses have now unequivocally shown superiority of PFO device closure over standard-of-care antithrombotic agents for all young patients (aged ≤60 years) with stroke of no other apparent cause other than PFO.[35–37,46–48] Moreover, the lessons learned from these studies have allowed the authors to extrapolate these data and apply them to their everyday patients, some of whom may have been neglected from the randomized studies.

Device-Associated Atrial Fibrillation: Protection from Patent Foramen Ovale-Mediated Stroke Only to Cause Another Stroke Etiology?

Percutaneous PFO closure has been associated with a 4-fold higher risk of new-onset atrial fibrillation,[62] which raises a reasonable concern whether this procedure, although decreasing the likelihood of PFO-mediated stroke recurrence, adds another thromboembolic stroke risk factor. It is highly reassuring that most of these new atrial arrhythmia events were consisted of a single isolated episode, occurred during or early (<30 days) after the procedure, and rarely led to a recurrent cerebrovascular event or required long-term anticoagulation. Only 5 out of 1889 (~0.1%) patients in all 6 trials developed recurrent stroke attributed to device-associated atrial fibrillation, and 3 of these cases were with the STARFlex device that is no longer commercially available.[17,64–66] Therefore, the stroke risk that this type of atrial fibrillation conveys seems to be minimal, and most of the patients do not require long-term anticoagulation (eg, 70% of the patients in CLOSE who developed device-associated atrial fibrillation eventually had their anticoagulation discontinued).[35–37,46–48] One observational study reported that only 3.8% of post-PFO closure atrial fibrillation cases progress to permanent atrial fibrillation.[67]

The Dangerous Patent Foramen Ovale: Device Closure for High-Risk Versus Low-Risk Patent Foramen Ovale

The recent RESPECT and REDUCE trials, which indiscriminately included all PFOs, showed that all young patients who suffer from stroke attributed to PFO will benefit from device closure over standard-of-care medical therapy on long-term follow-up.[41,46] Moreover, the randomized trials have also broadened the understanding of stroke patients who are found to have high-risk PFO features; both randomized and nonrandomized studies have demonstrated an even further enhanced clinical yield when device closure was performed for PFO associated with high-risk echocardiographic features (atrial septal aneurysm, hypermobile septum, Eustachian valve, Chiari network, or significant shunt through a large PFO).[41,47,48,68] For example, subanalyses of RESPECT demonstrated that when device closure was performed for high-risk PFO (atrial septal aneurysm or large shunt), there was a 3- to 4-fold lower rate of recurrent ischemic events when compared with blood thinners alone (P interaction = .04 for both).[41] The data from the CLOSE and DEFENSE-PFO studies, trials that only included high-risk PFOs, supported these findings, yielding 0 recurrent strokes in the device arm at 2 and 5 years, respectively (NNT = 10 and 20, respectively).[47,48] Even the strongest anticoagulant has yet to show such a therapeutic achievement for secondary stroke prevention, likewise considering the 2% to 4% annual bleeding risk of oral anticoagulation that increases with age. Intuitively, it makes clinical sense that a high-risk PFO would be more dangerous. A large PFO exhibits more right-to-left shunting; an atrial septal aneurysm or hypermobile septum will open the PFO with nearly every heartbeat, and a Eustachian valve or Chiari network will escort thrombi from the inferior vena cava straight to the PFO opening. Thus, a high-risk PFO may be considered an enhanced reason for device closure in these patients with ischemic stroke (Fig. 2).[17] However, it should be noted that in the REDUCE trial, the treatment effect of PFO closure did not differ based on PFO size (P interaction = .77). The enhanced effect with large PFOs seen in RESPECT should be considered hypothesis generating, and young ischemic stroke patients should not be deprived of the option of device therapy if a "small" PFO is seen on echocardiography.

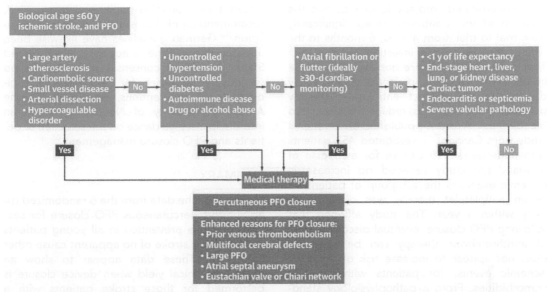

Fig. 2. Evidence-based algorithm for PFO closure in ischemic stroke patients for highest clinical yield, based on the randomized trials. (*From* Mojadidi et al. Cryptogenic Stroke and Patent Foramen Ovale: J Am Coll Cardiol; 2018;71(9):1035–43. Copyright © year 2018, with permission.)

Patent Foramen Ovale Device Closure for Elderly Patients with Stroke

Except for the DEFENSE-PFO study, elderly patients aged greater than 60 years were excluded from the randomized trials of PFO closure. These patients are more likely to have the traditional risk factors for stroke, including atherosclerosis, uncontrolled hypertension and diabetes, and atrial fibrillation. Recent randomized trials have shown that paroxysmal atrial fibrillation is underdiagnosed in elderly patients with ischemic stroke that is initially thought to be cryptogenic.[69,70] Thus, aggressively ruling out other causes of stroke, including occult atrial fibrillation with ≥30-day event monitoring, is recommended in these elderly patients.[71] However, it is also well known that paradoxical embolism is not a phenomenon that is restricted only to young patients.[65] There are stroke patients in their 60s or 70s with no evidence of atherosclerosis, atrial fibrillation, or other stroke causes; because PFO closure has an excellent safety profile, device closure may be considered for these patients, especially when associated with a high-risk PFO.[68]

Anticoagulation Versus Antiplatelet Therapy or Patent Foramen Ovale Closure

Although thromboembolism is considered the pathophysiology of PFO-mediated stroke, there remains a paucity of data comparing oral anticoagulation with PFO closure or antiplatelet therapy. The CLOSE trial was the only randomized study that had an oral anticoagulant, antiplatelet, and PFO closure arm; the study attempted to compare anticoagulation with antiplatelets. Although the trial demonstrated a nonsignificant 56% reduction in recurrent stroke with anticoagulation, the study was underpowered to make this comparison.[47] Current randomized data have not yet proven the superiority of warfarin or novel oral anticoagulants over antiplatelet therapy for prevention of recurrent embolic stroke of undetermined source,[72–74] even in the subset who have a PFO.[75,76] Until a randomized trial is completed that compares the efficacy and safety of percutaneous PFO closure with oral anticoagulation for secondary prevention of PFO-mediated stroke, percutaneous device closure should be considered the most effective therapy based on the current randomized data. Recently, a network meta-analysis proposed that patients receiving oral anticoagulation may have similar long-term stroke risk reduction as PFO closure.[77] However, experts give preference to device closure over oral anticoagulation given the better safety profile with PFO closure, including less risk of major bleeding, especially with a survival over decades that is typical for these younger patients.[78]

Patent Foramen Ovale Closure Plus Antiplatelet Therapy Versus Patent Foramen Ovale Closure Alone

In all 6 trials, PFO closure was combined with antiplatelet therapy in order to decrease the risk for device-related thrombotic events, but the duration of this treatment varied significantly from trial to trial (from at least 6 months to the whole duration of the investigation).[35–37,46–48] Therefore, the trials were not able to provide insight regarding the appropriate time to safely discontinue the adjunct antiplatelet therapy postprocedure and, thus, reduce the associated bleeding risk. A recently published observational study from Canada[79] investigated 453 patients who underwent PFO closure for a median of 8 years; the study revealed no increase in ischemic events in the subgroup of patients in whom antiplatelet therapy was discontinued early within a year. The study affirmed that following PFO closure, eventual discontinuation of antithrombotic therapy can be safe and does not appear to increase risk of recurrent ischemic events, for patients without other comorbidities. From a pathophysiology standpoint, it makes sense to complete 3 to 6 months of antiplatelet therapy following device closure, until complete endothelialization has occurred. Reported cases of intracerebral bleeding after PFO closure, when long-term antiplatelet therapy is continued,[68] reinforces the concept that indiscriminate continuation of such drugs after device closure may not be necessary.[79]

GUIDELINES FOR PATENT FORAMEN OVALE CLOSURE

The positive findings of the recently published stroke trials resulted in FDA approval of both the Amplatzer PFO Occluder and the Gore Cardioform Septal Occluder in October 2016 and March 2018, respectively.[45,80] The approvals are limited to use in patients generally aged 18 to 60 years old, with stroke attributed to paradoxical embolism by a neurologist and cardiologist.[45,80] The American Heart Association/American Stroke Association guidelines recommended medical treatment of secondary prevention of stroke in patients with PFO (class I recommendation), advising against device closure (class III recommendation).[81] However, these guidelines were issued in 2014 and have yet to be updated to reflect the most recent randomized data. The Heart and Stroke Foundation of Canada has already updated their guidelines as of November 2017, recommending PFO closure plus antiplatelet therapy for stroke prevention in young patients similar to the cohort studied in the clinical trials that led to approval of devices.[82] Likewise, various European organizations, including the European Stroke Organization and the European Society of Cardiology,

issued a joint position paper in January 2017, recommending PFO closure for the same population.[83] German guidelines have likewise been updated in the same direction.[84] In the United States, an expert consensus statement issued recently by the Society for Cardiovascular Angiography and Interventions, and affirmed by the American Academy of Neurology, offers an interdisciplinary guidance on the selection of patients and PFO closure management.[85]

SUMMARY

In summary, the data from the 6 randomized trials support percutaneous PFO closure for secondary stroke prevention in all young patients with ischemic stroke of no apparent cause other than PFO. These data appear to show an enhanced clinical yield when device closure is performed for those stroke patients with a high-risk PFO. Expert consensus groups recommend PFO closure as preferable to oral anticoagulation for these patients because of a better long-term safety profile, including less risk of major bleeding. Six randomized trials have shown that percutaneous PFO closure is safe, with a long-term safety profile that is similar to standard-of-care medical therapy. Device-associated atrial arrhythmias are a potential risk occurring in 4% to 5% of patients who receive a device; however, the data demonstrate that most of these cases occur early (less than 30 days), are transient (a single episode), and usually do not require long-term oral anticoagulation or pose a significant stroke risk.

There are several questions that need to be answered and challenges that need to be addressed in the future. First, elderly patients were excluded from the trials, and there is a paucity of observational data on the utility of PFO closure in these patients. It is common knowledge that paradoxical embolism is not a condition exclusive to young patients. Therefore, future trials recruiting well-selected elderly patients are needed to truly determine the efficacy and safety of PFO closure for these patients.[86] Second, the optimal duration of antiplatelet therapy in patients who have undergone PFO closure has not been examined by the trials, but there is evidence that early discontinuation does not increase the risk of stroke in otherwise healthy patients who do not have another indication for blood thinners. Third, now that the characteristics have been identified that make a PFO dangerous (ie, the high-risk PFO), is there a role of PFO closure for primary prevention in those patients, predominantly if they are also at high risk for venous thromboembolism? Screening and studying patients who are undergoing major surgery[87] and those with deep vein thrombosis or pulmonary embolism[88] would be a reasonable place to start looking. Finally, by proving that PFO closure decreases the risk of recurrent stroke, the recent trials confirmed the causal relationship between PFO and "cryptogenic stroke." Hence, it would be inappropriate to continue labeling PFO-mediated stroke[86] as "cryptogenic" in the face of this glaring culprit, because the misclassification continues to ignore the diagnostic and management strategies proposed by updated international guidelines and the FDA. PFO-associated stroke must be recognized as a unique and separate ischemic stroke entity when no other causes can be found. This change in terminology would be in line with the way paroxysmal atrial fibrillation- or flutter-mediated stroke was taken out of the heading of "cryptogenic stroke" and now widely accepted as a common cause of stroke.[71,89,90]

REFERENCES

1. Benjamin EJ, Blaha MJ, Chiuve SE, et al. Heart disease and stroke statistics—2017 update: a report from the American Heart Association. Circulation 2017;135(10):e146–603.
2. Lechat P, Mas JL, Lascault G, et al. Prevalence of patent foramen ovale in patients with stroke. N Engl J Med 1988;318(18):1148–52.
3. Hagen PT, Scholz DG, Edwards WD. Incidence and size of patent foramen ovale during the first 10 decades of life: an autopsy study of 965 normal hearts. Mayo Clin Proc 1984;59(1):17–20.
4. Webster MW, Chancellor AM, Smith HJ, et al. Patent foramen ovale in young stroke patients. Lancet 1988;2(8601):11–2.
5. Cohnheim J. Thrombose und embolie. In: Vorlesungen über Allgemeine Pathologie, vol. 1. Berlin: Hirschwald; 1877. p. 134.
6. Johnson B. Paradoxical embolism. J Clin Pathol 1951;4(3):316.
7. Crump R, Shandling AH, Van BN, et al. Prevalence of patent foramen ovale in patients with acute myocardial infarction and angiographically normal coronary arteries. Am J Cardiol 2000;85(11):1368–70.
8. Ward R, Jones D, Haponik EF. Paradoxical embolism: an underrecognized problem. Chest 1995;108(2):549–58.
9. De Castro S, Cartoni D, Fiorelli M, et al. Morphological and functional characteristics of patent foramen ovale and their embolic implications. Stroke 2000;31(10):2407–13.
10. Belkin RN, Hurwitz BJ, Kisslo J. Atrial septal aneurysm: association with cerebrovascular and peripheral embolic events. Stroke 1987;18(5):856–62.
11. Mas J-L, Arquizan C, Lamy C, et al. Recurrent cerebrovascular events associated with patent foramen ovale, atrial septal aneurysm, or both. N Engl J Med 2001;345(24):1740–6.
12. Schuchlenz HW, Saurer G, Weihs W, et al. Persisting Eustachian valve in adults: relation to patent foramen ovale and cerebrovascular events. J Am Soc Echocardiogr 2004;17(3):231–3.
13. Kato Y, Dembo T, Takeda H, et al. Prominent persisting Eustachian valve initiates spontaneous right-to-left shunt and paradoxical embolism in a patient with patent foramen ovale. Neurol Sci 2011;32(5):925–6.
14. Tobis JM, Charles A, Silberstein SD, et al. Percutaneous closure of patent foramen ovale in patients with migraine: The PREMIUM Trial. J Am Coll Cardiol 2017;70(22):2766–74.
15. Mattle HP, Evers S, Hildick-Smith D, et al. Percutaneous closure of patent foramen ovale in migraine with aura, a randomized controlled trial. Eur Heart J 2016;37(26):2029–36.
16. Mojadidi MK, Ruiz JC, Chertoff J, et al. Patent foramen ovale and hypoxemia. Cardiol Rev 2019;27(1): 34–40.
17. Mojadidi MK, Zaman MO, Elgendy IY, et al. Cryptogenic stroke and patent foramen ovale. J Am Coll Cardiol 2018;71(9):1035–43.
18. Moon R, Camporesi E, Kisslo J. Patent foramen ovale and decompression sickness in divers. Lancet 1989;333(8637):513–4.
19. Mojadidi MK, Bokhoor PI, Gevorgyan R, et al. Sleep apnea in patients with and without a right-to-left shunt. J Clin Sleep Med 2015;11(11):1299–304.
20. Mojadidi MK, Christia P, Salamon J, et al. Patent foramen ovale: unanswered questions. Eur J Intern Med 2015;26(10):743–51.
21. Mojadidi MK, Gevorgyan R, Noureddin N, et al. The effect of patent foramen ovale closure in patients with platypnea-orthodeoxia syndrome. Catheter Cardiovasc Interv 2015;86(4):701–7.
22. Khessali H, Mojadidi MK, Gevorgyan R, et al. The effect of patent foramen ovale closure on visual aura without headache or typical aura with migraine headache. JACC Cardiovasc Interv 2012; 5(6):682–7.
23. Bridges ND, Hellenbrand W, Latson L, et al. Transcatheter closure of patent foramen ovale after presumed paradoxical embolism. Circulation 1992; 86(6):1902–8.
24. Agarwal S, Bajaj NS, Kumbhani DJ, et al. Meta-analysis of transcatheter closure versus medical therapy for patent foramen ovale in prevention of recurrent neurological events after presumed paradoxical embolism. JACC Cardiovasc Interv 2012; 5(7):777–89.
25. Mahmoud AN, Elgendy IY, Agarwal N, et al. Identification and quantification of patent foramen ovale-

mediated shunts: echocardiography and transcranial Doppler. Interv Cardiol Clin 2017;6(4):495–504.

26. Meier B, Frank B, Wahl A, et al. Secondary stroke prevention: patent foramen ovale, aortic plaque, and carotid stenosis. Eur Heart J 2012;33(6):705–13.

27. Taramasso M, Nietlispach F, Maisano F, et al. Patent foramen ovale: indications for closure and techniques. EuroIntervention 2016;12(Suppl X):X7–x12.

28. Mojadidi MK, Bogush N, Caceres JD, et al. Diagnostic accuracy of transesophageal echocardiogram for the detection of patent foramen ovale: a meta-analysis. Echocardiography 2014;31(6):752–8.

29. Marchese N, Pacilli MA, Inchingolo V, et al. Residual shunt after percutaneous closure of patent foramen ovale with AMPLATZER occluder devices—influence of anatomic features: a transcranial Doppler and intracardiac echocardiography study. EuroIntervention 2013;9(3):382–8.

30. Mojadidi MK, Roberts SC, Winoker JS, et al. Accuracy of transcranial Doppler for the diagnosis of intracardiac right-to-left shunt: a bivariate meta-analysis of prospective studies. JACC Cardiovasc Imaging 2014;7(3):236–50.

31. Madala D, Zaroff JG, Hourigan L, et al. Harmonic imaging improves sensitivity at the expense of specificity in the detection of patent foramen ovale. Echocardiography 2004;21(1):33–6.

32. Mojadidi MK, Winoker JS, Roberts SC, et al. Accuracy of conventional transthoracic echocardiography for the diagnosis of intracardiac right-to-left shunt: a meta-analysis of prospective studies. Echocardiography 2014;31(9):1036–48.

33. Mojadidi MK, Winoker JS, Roberts SC, et al. Two-dimensional echocardiography using second harmonic imaging for the diagnosis of intracardiac right-to-left shunt: a meta-analysis of prospective studies. Int J Cardiovasc Imaging 2014;30(5):911–23.

34. Lamy C, Giannesini C, Zuber M, et al. Clinical and imaging findings in cryptogenic stroke patients with and without patent foramen ovale: the PFO-ASA Study. Stroke 2002;33(3):706–11.

35. Carroll JD, Saver JL, Thaler DE, et al. Closure of patent foramen ovale versus medical therapy after cryptogenic stroke. N Engl J Med 2013;368(12):1092–100.

36. Furlan AJ, Reisman M, Massaro J, et al. Closure or medical therapy for cryptogenic stroke with patent foramen ovale. N Engl J Med 2012;366(11):991–9.

37. Meier B, Kalesan B, Mattle HP, et al. Percutaneous closure of patent foramen ovale in cryptogenic embolism. N Engl J Med 2013;368(12):1083–91.

38. Hammerstingl C, Bauriedel B, Stusser C, et al. Risk and fate of residual interatrial shunting after transcatheter closure of patent foramen ovale: a long term follow up study. Eur J Med Res 2011;16(1):13–9.

39. Matsumura K, Gevorgyan R, Mangels D, et al. Comparison of residual shunt rates in five devices used to treat patent foramen ovale. Catheter Cardiovasc Interv 2014;84(3):455–63.

40. Mojadidi MK, Gevorgyan R, Tobis JM. Device closure of patent foramen ovale or medical therapy for cryptogenic stroke: the CLOSURE I trial. Patent foramen ovale. Springer; 2015. p. 173–9.

41. Saver JL, Carroll JD, Thaler DE, et al. Long-term outcomes of patent foramen ovale closure or medical therapy after stroke. N Engl J Med 2017;377(11):1022–32.

42. Rengifo-Moreno P, Palacios IF, Junpaparp P, et al. Patent foramen ovale transcatheter closure vs. medical therapy on recurrent vascular events: a systematic review and meta-analysis of randomized controlled trials. Eur Heart J 2013;34(43):3342–52.

43. Khan AR, Bin Abdulhak AA, Sheikh MA, et al. Device closure of patent foramen ovale versus medical therapy in cryptogenic stroke: a systematic review and meta-analysis. JACC Cardiovasc Interv 2013;6(12):1316–23.

44. Kent DM, Dahabreh IJ, Ruthazer R, et al. Device closure of patent foramen ovale after stroke: pooled analysis of completed randomized trials. J Am Coll Cardiol 2016;67(8):907–17.

45. Administration USFD. Premarket approval (PMA) 2016. Available at: https://www.accessdata.fda.gov/scripts/cdrh/cfdocs/cfpma/pma.cfm?id=P120021. Accessed March 20, 2019.

46. Sondergaard L, Kasner SE, Rhodes JF, et al. Patent foramen ovale closure or antiplatelet therapy for cryptogenic stroke. N Engl J Med 2017;377(11):1033–42.

47. Mas JL, Derumeaux G, Guillon B, et al. Patent foramen ovale closure or anticoagulation vs. antiplatelets after stroke. N Engl J Med 2017;377(11):1011–21.

48. Lee PH, Song JK, Kim JS, et al. Cryptogenic stroke and high-risk patent foramen ovale: the DEFENSE-PFO trial. J Am Coll Cardiol 2018;71(20):2335–42.

49. Palaiodimos L, Kokkinidis DG, Faillace RT, et al. Percutaneous closure of patent foramen ovale vs. medical treatment for patients with history of cryptogenic stroke: a systematic review and meta-analysis of randomized controlled trials. Cardiovasc Revasc Med 2018;19(7):852–8.

50. Kokkinidis D, Palaiodimos L, Faillace R, et al, editors. Percutaneous closure of patent foramen ovale vs. medical treatment for patients with history of cryptogenic stroke-a systematic review and meta-analysis of randomised controlled trials. Cerebrovascular Diseases. Basel (Switzerland): Karger; 2018.

51. Mojadidi MK, Elgendy AY, Elgendy IY, et al. Transcatheter patent foramen ovale closure after cryptogenic stroke: an updated meta-analysis of randomized trials. JACC Cardiovasc Interv 2017;10(21):2228–30.

52. Mojadidi MK, Mahmoud AN, Patel NK, et al. Cryptogenic stroke and patent foramen ovale: ready for prime time? J Am Coll Cardiol 2018;72(10):1183–5.

53. Ntaios G, Papavasileiou V, Sagris D, et al. Closure of patent foramen ovale versus medical therapy in patients with cryptogenic stroke or transient ischemic attack: updated systematic review and meta-analysis. Stroke 2018;49(2):412–8.

54. De Rosa S, Sievert H, Sabatino J, et al. Percutaneous closure versus medical treatment in stroke patients with patent foramen ovale: a systematic review and meta-analysis. Ann Intern Med 2018;168(5):343–50.

55. Abo-salem E, Chaitman B, Helmy T, et al. Patent foramen ovale closure versus medical therapy in cases with cryptogenic stroke, meta-analysis of randomized controlled trials. J Neurol 2018;265(3):578–85.

56. Shah R, Nayyar M, Jovin IS, et al. Device closure versus medical therapy alone for patent foramen ovale in patients with cryptogenic stroke: a systematic review and meta-analysis. Ann Intern Med 2018;168(5):335–42.

57. Vaduganathan M, Qamar A, Gupta A, et al. Patent foramen ovale closure for secondary prevention of cryptogenic stroke: updated meta-analysis of randomized clinical trials. Am J Med 2018;131(5):575–7.

58. Turc G, Calvet D, Guérin P, et al. Closure, anticoagulation, or antiplatelet therapy for cryptogenic stroke with patent foramen ovale: systematic review of randomized trials, sequential meta-analysis, and new insights from the CLOSE study. J Am Heart Assoc 2018;7(12):e008356.

59. Lattanzi S, Brigo F, Cagnetti C, et al. Patent foramen ovale and cryptogenic stroke or transient ischemic attack: to close or not to close? A systematic review and meta-analysis. Cerebrovasc Dis 2018;45(5–6):193–203.

60. Ahmad Y, Howard JP, Arnold A, et al. Patent foramen ovale closure vs. medical therapy for cryptogenic stroke: a meta-analysis of randomized controlled trials. Eur Heart J 2018;39(18):1638–49.

61. Riaz H, Khan MS, Schenone AL, et al. Transcatheter closure of patent foramen ovale following cryptogenic stroke: an updated meta-analysis of randomized controlled trials. Am Heart J 2018;199:44–50.

62. Kokkinidis DG, Palaiodimos L, Mastoris I, et al. The best DEFENSE for high-risk patent foramen ovale: an updated meta-analysis of six randomized trials. Arch Cardiovasc Dis 2018;112(3):150–2.

63. Verma SK, Tobis JM. Explantation of patent foramen ovale closure devices: a multicenter survey. JACC Cardiovasc Interv 2011;4(5):579–85.

64. Mojadidi MK, Elgendy AY, Elgendy IY, et al. Atrial fibrillation after percutaneous patent foramen ovale closure. Am J Cardiol 2018;122(5):915.

65. Ando T, Holmes AA, Pahuja M, et al. Meta-analysis comparing patent foramen ovale closure versus medical therapy to prevent recurrent cryptogenic stroke. Am J Cardiol 2018;121(5):649–55.

66. Elgendy A, Elgendy I, Mojadidi M, et al. New-onset atrial fibrillation following percutaneous patent foramen ovale closure: a systematic review and meta-analysis of randomised trials. EuroIntervention 2019;14(17):1788–90.

67. Staubach S, Steinberg DH, Zimmermann W, et al. New onset atrial fibrillation after patent foramen ovale closure. Catheter Cardiovasc Interv 2009;74(6):889–95.

68. Takafuji H, Hosokawa S, Ogura R, et al. Percutaneous transcatheter closure of high-risk patent foramen ovale in the elderly. Heart Vessels 2019;1–6.

69. Sanna T, Diener H-C, Passman RS, et al. Cryptogenic stroke and underlying atrial fibrillation. N Engl J Med 2014;370(26):2478–86.

70. Gladstone DJ, Spring M, Dorian P, et al. Atrial fibrillation in patients with cryptogenic stroke. N Engl J Med 2014;370(26):2467–77.

71. Hart RG, Diener H-C, Coutts SB, et al. Embolic strokes of undetermined source: the case for a new clinical construct. Lancet Neurol 2014;13(4):429–38.

72. Mohr JP, Thompson JL, Lazar RM, et al. A comparison of warfarin and aspirin for the prevention of recurrent ischemic stroke. N Engl J Med 2001;345(20):1444–51.

73. Hart RG, Sharma M, Mundl H, et al. Rivaroxaban for stroke prevention after embolic stroke of undetermined source. N Engl J Med 2018;378(23):2191–201.

74. TCTMD. Dabigatran trials come up short for stroke of unknown cause and cerebral venous thrombosis. 2018. Available at: https://www.tctmd.com/news/dabigatran-trials-come-short-stroke-unknown-cause-and-cerebral-venous-thrombosis. Accessed March 20, 2019.

75. Homma S, Sacco RL, Di Tullio MR, et al. Effect of medical treatment in stroke patients with patent foramen ovale: patent foramen ovale in Cryptogenic Stroke Study. Circulation 2002;105(22):2625–31.

76. Kasner SE, Swaminathan B, Lavados P, et al. Rivaroxaban or aspirin for patent foramen ovale and embolic stroke of undetermined source: a prespecified subgroup analysis from the NAVIGATE ESUS trial. Lancet Neurol 2018;17(12):1053–60.

77. Mir H, Siemieniuk RAC, Ge LC, et al. Patent foramen ovale closure, antiplatelet therapy or anticoagulation in patients with patent foramen ovale and cryptogenic stroke: a systematic review and network meta-analysis incorporating complementary external evidence. BMJ Open 2018;8(7):e023761.

78. Kuijpers T, Spencer FA, Siemieniuk RAC, et al. Patent foramen ovale closure, antiplatelet therapy or anticoagulation therapy alone for management of cryptogenic stroke? A clinical practice guideline. BMJ 2018;362:k2515.

79. Wintzer-Wehekind J, Alperi A, Houde C, et al. Impact of discontinuation of antithrombotic therapy following closure of patent foramen ovale in patients with cryptogenic embolism. Am J Cardiol 2019;123(9):1538–45.

80. Adminitration USFD. GORE® CARDIOFORM septal occluder - P050006/S060. 2018. Available at: https://www.fda.gov/MedicalDevices/ProductsandMedical-Procedures/DeviceApprovalsandClearances/Recently-ApprovedDevices/ucm604786.htm. Accessed March 20, 2019.

81. Kernan WN, Ovbiagele B, Black HR, et al. Guidelines for the prevention of stroke in patients with stroke and transient ischemic attack: a guideline for healthcare professionals from the American Heart Association/American Stroke Association. Stroke 2014;45(7):2160–236.

82. Wein T, Lindsay MP, Côté R, et al. Canadian stroke best practice recommendations: secondary prevention of stroke, practice guidelines, update 2017. Int J Stroke 2018;13(4):420–43.

83. Pristipino C, Sievert H, D'Ascenzo F, et al. European position paper on the management of patients with patent foramen ovale. General approach and left circulation thromboembolism. Eur Heart J 2018. [Epub ahead of print].

84. DGN. Leitlinien für Diagnostik_und_Therapie_in der_Neurologie. 2018. Available at: https://www.dgn.org/46-startseite/3642-ende-des-patts-kardiologen-und-neurologen-empfehlen-pfo-verschluss-zum-schutz-vor-schlaganfall. Accessed March 20, 2019.

85. Horlick E, Kavinsky CJ, Amin Z, et al. SCAI expert consensus statement on operator and institutional requirements for PFO closure for secondary prevention of paradoxical embolic stroke: the American Academy of Neurology affirms the value of this statement as an educational tool for neurologists. Catheter Cardiovasc Interv 2019;93(5):859–74.

86. Zaman MO, Patel NK, Mojadidi MK. Patent foramen ovale closure for patients excluded from the randomized cryptogenic stroke trials. Clin Res Cardiol 2018;107(12):1187–8.

87. Ng PY, Ng AK-Y, Subramaniam B, et al. Association of preoperatively diagnosed patent foramen ovale with perioperative ischemic stroke. JAMA 2018;319(5):452–62.

88. Konstantinides S, Geibel A, Kasper W, et al. Patent foramen ovale is an important predictor of adverse outcome in patients with major pulmonary embolism. Circulation 1998;97(19):1946–51.

89. Adams H Jr, Bendixen B, Kappelle L, et al. Trial of Org 10172 in Acute Stroke Treatment. Classification of subtype of acute ischemic stroke: definitions for use in a multicenter clinical trial. Stroke 1993;24(1):35–41.

90. Amarenco P, Bogousslavsky J, Caplan L, et al. The ASCOD phenotyping of ischemic stroke (Updated ASCO Phenotyping). Cerebrovasc Dis 2013;36(1):1–5.

Adjunct Pharmacotherapy After Transcatheter Aortic Valve Replacement
Current Status and Future Directions

David A. Power, MBBCh[a], Paul Guedeney, MD[b],
George D. Dangas, MD, PhD[a],*

KEYWORDS
• TAVR • Antiplatelet • SAPT • DAPT • Oral anticoagulation • Antithrombotic

KEY POINTS
• Although transcatheter aortic valve replacement (TAVR) is a validated treatment option for severe aortic valve stenosis, few randomized data exist to guide the optimal antithrombotic strategy in the postprocedural period. • Single or dual antiplatelet therapy (SAPT or DAPT), with or without oral anticoagulation (OAC) have emerged as possible treatment strategies after TAVR. • Existing guidelines from scientific societies are mostly based on expert opinion, and considerable variation in practices exist regarding post-TAVR antithrombotic therapy. • SAPT may be safer than DAPT in patients at bleeding risk who do not have atrial fibrillation, although larger randomized controlled trials are required for definitive answers. • OACs with or without SAPT may be reasonable options in patients with atrial fibrillation; randomized clinical trials are exploring this subject.

INTRODUCTION

Transcatheter aortic valve replacement (TAVR) is an increasingly common intervention for patients with severe symptomatic aortic stenosis (AS). TAVR has become validated as the standard of care for patients with symptomatic AS at high and intermediate surgical risk profiles.[1,2] Expansion of its indication is anticipated in low-risk patients based on clinical trial results.[3,4] Since the end of 2017, it is estimated that over 300,000 aortic valve replacements have been performed via the less invasive transcatheter approach.[5]

In the United States, the prevalence of calcific AS is expected to grow alongside an aging patient demographic, and therefore the number of TAVR procedures is expected to continue growing rapidly. Ischemic, embolic, and bleeding events have remained important complications since the emergence of TAVR. Clarifying the safest and most effective postprocedural antithrombotic regimen to balance bleeding and ischemic risk in these patients is therefore critical.[6,7]

The optimal intensity and duration of antithrombotic therapy for the prevention of ischemic

Disclosure: D.A. Power and P. Guedeney have nothing to disclose. G.D. Dangas is a consultant to Bayer, Janssen Pharmaceuticals, Inc, Daiichi-Sankyo; a Scientific Advisor to AstraZeneca; has equity in Claret Medical Inc; and has received a research grant to the institution from Bayer and Daiichi-Sankyo.
[a] The Zena and Michael A. Wiener Cardiovascular Institute, Icahn School of Medicine at Mount Sinai, One Gustave L. Levy Place, Box 1030, New York City, NY 10029, USA; [b] ACTION Coeur, Sorbonne Université, UMR_S 1166, Institut de Cardiologie (APHP), Hôpital Pitié Salpêtrière, 47-83 Boulevard de l'Hôpital, Paris 75013, France
* Corresponding author.
E-mail address: george.dangas@mountsinai.org

Intervent Cardiol Clin 8 (2019) 357–371
https://doi.org/10.1016/j.iccl.2019.05.003
2211-7458/19/© 2019 Elsevier Inc. All rights reserved.

events after TAVR has not been clearly defined. Significant discordance exists among the clinical practice recommendations of major international guidelines and consensus documents.[1,2,8–10] In addition, different valve manufacturers suggest varying dosages and durations of postprocedural antithrombotic therapy in their respective "instructions for use" packaging.[11] The randomized trials that established TAVR as an alternative therapeutic approach to surgical intervention have also used different regimens of postprocedural medical therapies.[12–14]

In this review of adjunct pharmacotherapy after TAVR we explore the pathobiological rationale underlying post-TAVR antithrombotic therapy, examine the current evidence and major societal guidelines, and outline the major ongoing randomized controlled trials (RCTs) investigating antithrombotic regimens after TAVR. Finally, we attempt to reconcile the current recommendations and evidence to provide a pragmatic, evidence-based strategy for post-TAVR pharmacotherapy.

PATHOPHYSIOLOGY OF POSTTRANSCATHETER AORTIC VALVE REPLACEMENT COMPLICATIONS

Despite iterative improvements in valve design and procedural technique, ischemic and bleeding complications after TAVR remain frequent and have been associated with increased morbidity and mortality.[15] Valvular dysfunction following TAVR is related to a complex interplay between clinical, mechanical, pharmacologic, and biological factors. This dysfunction may cause reduced leaflet motion, impaired coaptation, leaflet thickening, altered effective orifice area, and increased transvalvular gradients or regurgitation.[16,17] Indeed, all foreign bodies implanted within the human cardiovascular system are potentially thrombogenic, thus implying a potential benefit with antithrombotic therapy.[18]

Transcatheter Valvular Implantation

The insertion of a valvular prosthesis without removal of the native calcified aortic valve creates an irregular zone around the valvular frame (a "neo-sinus") with turbulent and often low shear flow patterns that may predispose to fibrin deposition, thrombus formation, and embolization beyond the processes involved in normal healing.[19] Stenotic aortic valve leaflets are rich in tissue factor that can be locally exposed to circulating blood when they are disrupted. Longer-term data from bioprosthetic valve studies have suggested that the neointimal tissue growth and endothelialization of the valve stent probably occur about 3 months after implantation.[20,21] This is consistent with previous studies demonstrating that thromboembolic events are greatest within the first 3 months of implantation.[22] The pathobiological rationale behind post-TAVR antithrombotic therapy, therefore, focuses on protecting the implanted vascular prosthesis while the process of valve endothelialization is occurring. These overlapping factors would appear to support a more aggressive up-front period of antithrombotic therapy, followed by a maintenance therapy, similar to the paradigm of coronary stent implantation.[23] The antithrombotic and anti-ischemic effects associated with prolonged antithrombotic therapy are achieved at the expense of increased bleeding risk, which may be associated with increased morbidity and mortality.[7]

Bioprosthetic Valve Thrombosis

A broad spectrum of pathologic conditions related to transcatheter aortic valve thrombosis has been described. These can be classified and may range from incidental findings to severe obstructive valve thrombosis with congestive heart failure.[24–26] Studies have suggested that subclinical valve thrombosis may occur more frequently in transcatheter valves compared with the bioprosthetic valves implanted through the traditional open surgical approach.[27] The diagnostic criteria for bioprosthetic valve thrombosis are based primarily on 4-dimensional computerized tomographic angiography findings: specifically a new hemodynamic deterioration (increase in mean transprosthetic gradient and/or worsening or new intraprosthetic regurgitation), increased leaflet thickness, reduced leaflet motion/coaptation, and a favorable response to antithrombotic therapy.[28] Only at rather advanced stages may there be clear echocardiographic findings.[29,30]

Bleeding

In terms of bleeding risk, important differentiating characteristics exist between coronary stents and transcatheter valves, given differences in patient characteristics (eg, age) and procedural characteristics (eg, large-bore femoral arterial access for valve delivery).[31] The need for large-bore arteriotomy access potentiates the risk of early bleeding with the use of antithrombotic agents, particularly when combined with periprocedural antiplatelet loading regimens. In this regard, the use of preprocedural dual antiplatelet therapy (DAPT) has been associated with an increased risk of bleeding. Following the procedure, the risk of major bleeding progressively decreases over time, particularly from vascular access sites. Importantly, nonaccess site bleeding has been previously shown to be most significantly associated with post-TAVR mortality.[32] However, the impact of these medications on bleeding has not been tracked carefully and may vary substantially with types of medications after TAVR.

Although the risk of ischemic cerebrovascular events declines after approximately 3 months postprocedure, the risk of stroke has been previously shown to extend to 1 year. The risk of thromboembolism, therefore, extends beyond the procedure itself and persists throughout early follow-up. Overall, the pathophysiology of transcatheter valve implantation, valve thrombosis, and bleeding complications illustrates the complex interplay and risk-benefit tradeoffs associated with antithrombotic therapies following TAVR (Fig. 1).

CEREBROVASCULAR COMPLICATIONS AFTER TRANSCATHETER AORTIC VALVE REPLACEMENT

The rates of stroke following TAVR have remained relatively unchanged until recently.[15,33] Analysis of the PARTNER-2 (placement of aortic transcatheter valves 2) intermediate-risk trial showed an increased risk of stroke at 30 days (5.5%) and 12 months (8.0%).[12] These patients are typically elderly, with multiple comorbidities.[34] Periprocedural anticoagulation and intraprocedural embolic protection devices have been possible preventative strategies for perioperative stroke prevention.[35] Recently, the PARTNER-3 low-risk trial showed a significant improvement in rates of stroke following TAVR, with a 30-day stroke

rate of 0.6% and 12-month rate of 1.2%.[3] However, given the aforementioned risk profile of the PARTNER-2 population, a clearer understanding of the risk-benefit profile of mid- to long-term antithrombotic strategies are of paramount importance. The relation of ischemic and thrombotic events after TAVR can be classified (acute, subacute, and late) with varying causes of cerebrovascular accidents according to the timing of the event[36] (Fig. 2).

Silent cerebral embolization following TAVR is a relatively common occurrence. MRI studies have shown that subclinical cerebrovascular insults are frequent.[36,37] On the other hand, clinically overt stroke following TAVR in patients with intermediate-to-high surgical risk ranges from 1% to 3% within the first 30 days and averages 4% to 5% at 1 year.[15] Strokes occurring within the periprocedural and acute phases (<24 hours) are predominantly related to technical and procedural factors. Clinically overt stroke occurring after this time period most likely relates to other longstanding pathophysiological factors, such as atrial fibrillation (AF), prosthetic valve thrombosis, and atherothrombotic disease.[38,39] In a study examining the embolic debris captured by protection devices during TAVR, approximately 3 out of 4 patients had macroscopically visible debris. When examining the nature of the embolic debris, approximately half (55%) of patients had thrombotic debris, with 70% having matter consistent with degenerative aortic valve tissue or aortic wall fragments.[38,40] Given the significant morbidity and mortality associated with postprocedural clinical stroke following TAVR, this is an important area for further clinical study and characterization of risks and therapeutic benefit.

The clinical significance of clinically "silent" ischemic or embolic events associated with

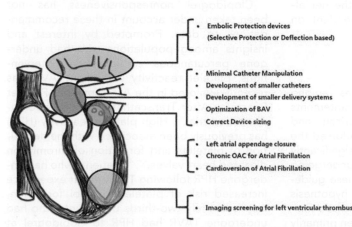

- Embolic Protection devices
  (Selective Protection or Deflection based)

- Minimal Catheter Manipulation
- Development of smaller catheters
- Development of smaller delivery systems
- Optimization of BAV
- Correct Device sizing

- Left atrial appendage closure
- Chronic OAC for Atrial Fibrillation
- Cardioversion of Atrial Fibrillation

- Imaging screening for left ventricular thrombus

Fig. 1. Selected cerebrovascular protection strategies for TAVR. BAV, balloon aortic valvuloplasty; OAC, oral anticoagulant. (*Data from* Giustino G, Dangas G. Stroke prevention in valvular heart disease: from the procedure to long-term management. Eurointervention. 2015;11(W):W26-W31; with permission.)

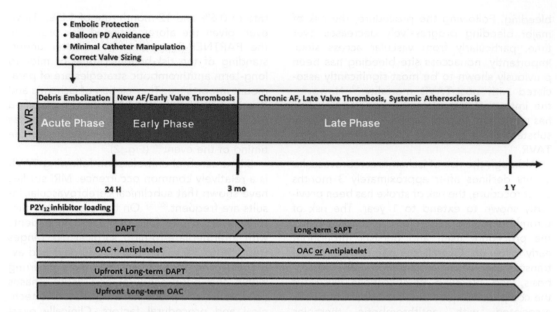

Fig. 2. Timeline of early and late stroke complications with selected antithrombotic pharmacotherapies. AF, atrial fibrillation; DAPT, dual antiplatelet therapy; OAC, oral anticoagulant; PD, postdilation; SAPT, single antiplatelet therapy; TAVR, transcatheter aortic valvular replacement. Note: P2Y$_{12}$ inhibitor loading is not standardized and controversial.

TAVR is not fully understood. Although some cardiothoracic surgery studies have found steeper declines in cognitive function and increased rates of dementia following valve implantation, 1 study examining patients who had undergone TAVR with new clinically silent lesions found that only 5% had early cognitive decline.[41,42] In contrast, a prospective study of approximately 50 patients demonstrated improved cognitive abilities following TAVR; this effect was more pronounced in those with cognitive impairment at baseline, suggesting particular benefit with this group.[43] It is possible that the enhanced circulatory effects after TAVR may portend a benefit, and embolization the opposite: hence, the net effect on each patient may be dependent on both.

SUMMARY OF GUIDELINES

There are considerable differences among the current cardiovascular consensus statements and guidelines. The major American and European recommendations have endorsed the use of DAPT in the absence of a significantly increased bleeding risk for patients undergoing TAVR. It is important to note that these guidelines were originally based on the hypothesis that bioprosthetic valves "ought to behave similarly" to coronary stents and are driven primarily

by expert opinion, rather than qualifying randomized trials.[1,2,8,9]

The 2014 and the 2017 update of the American Heart Associated/American College of Cardiology (AHA/ACC) guidelines on valvular heart disease suggest lifelong aspirin plus 6 months of clopidogrel "may be reasonable" following transcatheter valve implantation. This recommendation is IIb, level of evidence C; indicating that the recommendation is driven by expert opinion with limited evidence. The 2017 ACC Expert Consensus Document proposes a current standard antithrombotic therapy after TAVR with lifelong aspirin and 3 to 6 months of therapy with oral clopidogrel.[2,44]

Clopidogrel nonresponsiveness has not been taken under account in these recommendations to date. Prompted by interest and insights among populations who had undergone percutaneous cardiovascular interventions, platelet reactivity testing in TAVR was recently explored in the Assessment of Platelet Reactivity After Transcatheter Aortic Valve Implantation trial.[45] High platelet reactivity (HPR) has previously been associated with the deposition of platelets and formation of thrombi on diseased heart valves.[46,47] Patients who had undergone HPR following TAVR might experience increased risk of platelet thrombi formation. Approximately two-thirds of patients who had undergone TAVR had HPR to clopidogrel at baseline.[48] Furthermore, over a third of patients initially identified as clopidogrel responders later developed HPR status during the first month after TAVR. The authors also found that ticagrelor effectively reduced HPR with consistent effects throughout the treatment period.[45] As of yet, however, there is a paucity of data linking HPR to clinical outcomes after TAVR. Therefore, there is insufficient evidence to advise routine HPR testing among patients undergoing TAVR. The relation between platelet reactivity and bleeding risk after TAVR should also be evaluated in future clinical trials.

The European Society of Cardiology (ESC) guidelines on valvular heart disease recommend that a combination of low-dose aspirin combined with a $P2Y_{12}$ inhibitor should be used early after TAVR, followed by monotherapy with either low-dose aspirin or a thienopyridine alone. The ESC does not, however, delineate specific antiplatelet durations following TAVR.[1] The Canadian Cardiovascular Society recommendation differ further—advising DAPT for 1 to 3 months, followed by antiplatelet monotherapy.[9] Finally, the American College of Cardiology Foundation/American Association for Thoracic Surgery/Society for Cardiovascular Angiography and Interventions/Society of Thoracic Surgeon recommend DAPT for 3 to 6 months following TAVR.[8] It is a widely accepted practice to empirically use DAPT, typically with clopidogrel and aspirin. However, this approach lacks evidence and has been adopted primarily on the example of coronary stent implantation where a dedicated period of DAPT is mandatory to prevent device thrombosis. A summary of the current guidelines is presented in Table 1 and Fig. 3.

Given the evident lack of unity among the major guidelines for antithrombotic therapy, it comes of little surprise that significant differences exist in individual prescribing practices. Wide discrepancies have been demonstrated in previous studies qualitatively and quantitatively examining the prescribing habits of TAVR operators.[11] These studies have demonstrated that most postprocedural therapies are predominately based on institutional policy or personal preference, rather than societal guidelines. Although valve manufacturers provide individual recommendations for antithrombotic therapy following valve implantation, a valve-specific approach to postprocedural antithrombotic therapy seems to be an uncommon practice.[49]

SINGLE ANTIPLATELET THERAPY VERSUS DUAL ANTIPLATELET THERAPY STRATEGIES

Stemming from the experience of intracoronary stents, the first trials evaluating TAVR used a DAPT strategy for up to 6 months with aspirin and clopidogrel as an antiplatelet regimen after valvular implantation.[10] This was born out of the idea of preventing bioprosthetic valve-related thrombotic complications while neointimal tissue growth and endothelialization of the metallic valve frame are ongoing.[19] Although DAPT following TAVR initially seemed to be a reasonably pragmatic strategy, it has been recently questioned because important tradeoffs in terms of bleeding associated with DAPT have been progressively realized. Similar to ongoing debate surrounding the risk-benefits and tradeoffs within percutaneous coronary stenting literature, Patients who had undergone TAVR remain at increased risk of bleeding.[23] There are important differences in the thrombotic tendencies of implanted TAVR valves compared with intracoronary stents, most notably the rather large size (approximately 10 times greater diameter of a valve vs stent) and bioprosthetic transcatheter valve design. In addition, the bleeding profiles of these patients is inherently altered, particularly given the necessity for large-bore arteriotomy sites. Hence, several TAVR trials have begun to examine the risk-benefit tradeoff of DAPT.[27,50–52]

The recommendations included within the original landmark PARTNER trial consisted of low-dose aspirin (75–100 mg) with clopidogrel (600 mg loading dose, followed by 75 mg daily) for 6 months after TAVR.[14] Several observational studies suggested that DAPT may the lack any important effect over SAPT for prevention of cerebrovascular events after TAVR.[53] At present, this paradigm of DAPT versus SAPT has been examined in only 3 small RCTs and a patient-level meta-analysis, albeit with small sample size.[54–56] The Aspirin Versus Aspirin + Clopidogrel Following TAVR trial, for example, randomized 222 patients who had undergone TAVR to 3 months of SAPT (daily low-dose aspirin) or DAPT (aspirin plus clopidogrel). Consistent with previous findings from observational studies, it showed a trend toward increased overall complications with DAPT (odds ratio [OR] = 2.31; 95% CI, 0.95–5.62; $P = .065$) compared with SAPT; major/life-threatening bleeding was increased 3-fold with DAPT (OR = 3.22; 95% CI, 1.01–10.34; $P = .038$) compared with SAPT.[54] The previously

Table 1
TAVR guideline summaries of antithrombotic therapy

TAVR Guidelines/Expert Consensus	Patients *Without* Underlying Indication for OAC	Patients *with* Underlying Indication for OAC
American College of Cardiology/American Heart Association 2017 Updated Recommendations[2]	Anticoagulation with a VKA to achieve an international normalized ratio of 2.5 may be reasonable in patients at low risk of bleeding for at least 3 mo *(IIb – B NR)* Clopidogrel 75 mg the first 6 mo after TAVR may be reasonable in addition to lifelong aspirin 75–100 mg daily *(IIb – C)*	No specific recommendations
European Society of Cardiology/European Association for Cardio-Thoracic Surgery 2017 Guidelines[1]	DAPT should be considered for the first 3–6 mo after TAVR, followed by lifelong SAPT in patients who do not need OAC for other reasons. *(IIa – C)* SAPT may be considered after TAVR in the case of high bleeding risk. *(IIb – C)*	Despite the lack of evidence, a combination of VKA and aspirin or thienopyridine is generally used but should be weighed against increased risk of bleeding. *(EC)*
American College of Cardiology Foundation/American Association for Thoracic Surgery/Society for Cardiovascular Angiography and Interventions/Society of Thoracic Surgeons 2012 Expert Consensus[8]	Antiplatelet therapy for at least 3–6 mo after TAVR is recommended to decrease the risk of thrombotic or thromboembolic complications. *(EC)*	In patients treated with warfarin, a direct thrombin inhibitor, or factor Xa inhibitor, it is reasonable to continue low-dose aspirin but other antiplatelet therapy should be avoided if possible. *(EC)*
Canadian Cardiovascular Society 2012 Position Statement[9]	In general, indefinite low-dose aspirin is recommended along with 1–3 mo of a thienopyridine. *(EC)*	The need for adjunctive antiplatelet agents is controversial, and triple therapy should be avoided unless definite indications exist. *(EC)*

mentioned HPR issue may also attenuate the SAPT versus DAPT differences.

Although insufficient to allow a definite conclusion regarding a best post-TAVR antithrombotic duration and agent, these data supported an equipoise and in fact led to a change in the 2017 ESC recommendations. In patients with high bleeding risk, SAPT may now be considered (class IIb).[1] Loading doses of P2Y$_{12}$ inhibitors (typically clopidogrel 600 mg), as recommended by the designers of the PARTNER trials, have not been specifically addressed within the guidelines.[3,12,14] In a recent study, antiplatelet loading before TAVR did not seem to offer any important benefits compared with no antiplatelet loading in terms of major adverse cardiovascular events, major bleeding, or major vascular complications.[57]

Increased rates of 30-day major or life-threatening bleeding have been associated with DAPT compared with SAPT. Most of these bleeding events occur within the first 48 hours and are typically related to transcatheter vascular access or pericardial complications.[58] This questions the need for pretreatment with DAPT, including loading dose clopidogrel, before the procedure. The Optimized Transcatheter Valvular Intervention registry showed that

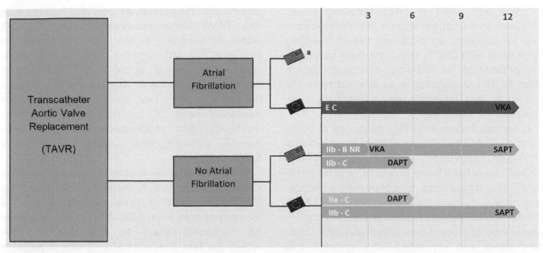

Fig. 3. Guideline comparison between ACC/AHA 2017 and ESC/EACTS 2017 on antithrombotic therapy following TAVR. DAPT, dual antiplatelet therapy; EC, Expert Consensus; SAPT, single antiplatelet therapy; VKA, vitamin K antagonist. [a] No guideline recommendations. (*Data from* Baumgartner H, Falk V, Bax JJ, et al. 2017 ESC/EACTS Guidelines for the management of valvular heart disease. European heart journal. 2017;38(36):2739-2791; and Nishimura Rick A, Otto Catherine M, Bonow Robert O, et al. 2017 AHA/ACC Focused Update of the 2014 AHA/ACC Guideline for the Management of Patients With Valvular Heart Disease: A Report of the American College of Cardiology/American Heart Association Task Force on Clinical Practice Guidelines. Circulation. 2017;135(25):e1159-e1195.)

pretreatment with DAPT was independently associated with increased in-hospital bleeding (OR = 2.05; 95% CI, 1.16–3.65).[59] These results have been replicated by other studies.[60] Given that over half of embolic protection devices seem to captured thrombotic debris—presumably related to perturbation of Virchow's triad—the impact of periprocedural DAPT loading on short-term and long-term outcomes requires ongoing study.

Several study-level meta-analyses have attempted to compare SAPT versus DAPT following TAVR.[11,61,62] Fernandes Gilson and colleagues,[61] in their meta-analysis of 691 patients treated with SAPT or DAPT following TAVR, showed no significant differences between treatment regimens at 30 days (OR = 0.88, 95% CI, 0.49–1.58; P = .67) and between 3 and 12 months (OR = 0.79, 95% CI, 0.45–1.38; P = .41). Rates of life-threatening and major bleeding were significantly lower in the SAPT group for short-term (OR = 0.37, 95% CI, 0.16–0.88; P = .02) and long-term follow-up (OR = 0.47, 95% CI, 0.25–0.90; P = .02). Additional meta-analyses of SAPT versus DAPT have all shown similar outcomes, DAPT being associated with an increased risk of major bleeding without benefit on overall mortality, stroke, or myocardial infarction after TAVR.[63] Although too early to make a definitive recommendation given limited data, initial results seem to suggest a

signal toward harm associated with DAPT after TAVR.[61]

Valve imaging studies have also assessed the role of DAPT versus SAPT in terms of their effects on rates of valve thrombosis. With increasing surveillance imaging quality after TAVR with computed tomography or transesophageal echocardiography, higher than expected rates of asymptomatic leaflet thrombosis are being detected.[27,64] The phenomenon of increased valve leaflet thrombosis (decreased leaflet mobility) may affect approximately 10% of patients within the first few months following TAVR and has, intuitively, been associated with an increased risk of stroke or transient ischemic attack.[65] There has been no differences in the prevalence of hypoattenuated leaflet thickening in patients treated with SAPT versus DAPT.[66,67] It is unclear whether thrombi produced during and after TAVR are of platelet or thrombin in origin, because the latter may not favor DAPT as an effective treatment modality. The previously mentioned tissue factor exposure theory certainly concurs.

DAPT is also indicated for those patients who had undergone TAVR with concomitant obstructive coronary artery disease treated with stenting, in keeping with the more definitive guidelines for antithrombotic therapy after percutaneous coronary intervention.[68] Overall, given the lack of randomized data, equipoise exists over whether to treat with DAPT or SAPT following TAVR. Although limited, the preponderance of evidence thus far suggests an increased risk of bleeding associated with DAPT, without a clear benefit in the prevention of ischemic events or death. Most RCTs are ongoing in an attempt to tackle this issue; thus far none uses a definitive, well-powered methodology.

In terms of alternative regimens, oral anticoagulation (OAC) with either vitamin K antagonists (VKA) or non-vitamin K oral anticoagulants (NOAC) have both been shown to treat and prevent leaflet thrombosis, thus providing an important clinical therapeutic mechanism after TAVR. In addition to the inherent differences in pathophysiology of thrombosis associated with coronary stents and implanted valve systems, this raises the important question of a potential benefit with anticoagulant therapy over antiplatelet therapy.[69] At the same time, possible bleeding complications with OAC must be considered.

Given the high risk of new-onset AF, subclinical leaflet thrombosis and overall ischemic events following TAVR, the systematic use of NOAC in patients without previous AF was hypothesized to be superior than the current DAPT-based strategy. The Global Study Comparing a Rivaroxaban-based Antithrombotic Strategy to an Antiplatelet-based Strategy After Transcatheter Aortic Valve Replacement to Optimize Clinical Outcomes trial (NCT02556203) evaluated this hypothesis by comparing rivoroxaban 10 mg daily plus low-dose aspirin versus DAPT (clopidogrel and aspirin) in patients without previous AF after TAVR (both arms drop an antiplatelet after 3 months). The trial was stopped owing to a higher risk of major adverse events in the rivoroxaban arm. At interim analysis, there was a higher rate of death or first thromboembolic event (11.4% vs 8.8%), all-cause death (6.8% vs 3.3%), and bleeding (4.2% vs 2.4%) with the rivoraxaban strategy.[33] Detailed results are expected to be presented later in 2019.[70]

ORAL ANTICOAGULATION AFTER TRANSCATHETER AORTIC VALVE REPLACEMENT

Approximately 1 in 3 patients who undergo TAVR have concomitant AF.[71] This presents an important clinical challenge for antithrombotic therapy following TAVR given the requirement for anticoagulation to prevent embolic events, in addition to weighing the risk of bleeding and having adequate therapy to prevent valve thrombosis. New-onset AF may also be common after TAVR with an incidence approaching 15% within 30 days and as much as 25% within the first year.[72–74] Although this is significantly lower than after surgical aortic valve replacement (SAVR), it remains a sizable subset of patients. Importantly, AF has been associated with increased rates of postprocedural mortality, morbidity, and readmission compared with non-AF patients who undergo TAVR and SAVR.[75,76]

Robust evidence supporting current antithrombotic strategies in these patients requiring OAC after TAVR is quite limited. The 2017 focused update from ACC/AHA provides a level IIB recommendation to the use of VKA within the first 3 months after TAVR in patients without high risk of bleeding.[2,44] Such recommendations were mostly based from the troubling findings by 4-dimensional volume-rendered computed tomography (4DCT) scan-based studies. The Subclinical Aortic Valve Bioprosthesis Thrombosis Assessed with Four-Dimensional Computed Tomography and the Assessment of Transcatheter and Surgical Aortic Bioprosthetic Valve Thrombosis and Its Treatment with Anticoagulation registries reported the presence of subclinical leaflet thrombosis in 13%. The presence of hypoattenuated leaflet thickening and/or reduced leaflet motion, which has been used to define the presence of subclinical leaflet thrombosis, has been associated with an increased risk of cerebrovascular events.[27,77]

The guidelines do not make recommendations regarding the use of NOACs for patients with AF undergoing TAVR. NOACs have demonstrated a more favorable efficacy and safety ratio compared with VKA for the prevention of thromboembolic complications of AF in other settings, and one could hypothesize that these qualities might be maintained in the setting of TAVR.[78,79] Early data of NOACs after TAVR in patients with AF, however, remain scarce and are derived mainly from observational registries. A single-center study of 617 patients undergoing TAVR suggested an association with apixaban and improved safety outcomes, compared with VKA, in patients with AF. The composite 30-day safety outcome occurred in 13.5% of apixaban patients compared with 30.5% of patients who received VKA ($P<.01$), driven predominantly by lower rates of acute kidney injury (2.1% vs 8.4%, $P<.01$) and life-threatening bleeding (3.5% vs 5.3%, $P<.01$).[80,81] The FRANCE-TAVI investigators, in their national prospective registry, examined outcomes and the occurrence of bioprosthetic valve

Table 2
Key randomized trials evaluating antithrombotic regimens after TAVR

	Trial	Antithrombotic Regimen	Treatment Duration	Target Enrollment	Anticipated Completion
No indication for OAC	GALILEO[70] (Global Study Comparing a Rivaroxaban-based Antithrombotic Strategy to an Antiplatelet-based Strategy After Transcatheter Aortic Valve Replacement to Optimize Clinical Outcomes) NCT02556203	Rivaroxaban 10 mg & acetylsalicylic acid (ASA) × 3 mo vs DAPT × 3 mo	ASA stopped or clopidogrel stopped after 3 mo, respectively	1644	Trial stopped due to safety concerns with the Rivaroxaban arm. Final results pending
	AUREA (Dual Antiplatelet Therapy vs Oral Anticoagulation for a Short Time to Prevent Cerebral Embolism After TAVI) NCT01642134	ASA & clopidogrel vs VKA	3 mo	124	2019
Indication for OAC	AVATAR (Anticoagulation Alone vs Anticoagulation and Aspirin Following Transcatheter Aortic Valve Interventions) NCT02735902	Aspirin + VKA vs VKA	12 mo	312	April 2020
	ENVISAGE-TAVI AF[88] (Edoxaban Compared to Standard Care After Heart Valve Replacement Using a Catheter in Patients with Atrial Fibrillation) NCT02943785	Edoxaban vs VKA	Until endpoint reached	1400	November 2020

(continued on next page)

Trial	Antithrombotic Regimen	Treatment Duration	Target Enrollment	Anticipated Completion
With and without indication for OAC				
POPular-TAVI[87] (Antiplatelet Therapy for Patients Undergoing Transcatheter Aortic Valve Implantation) NCT02247128	ASA vs DAPT or VKA vs VKA & clopidogrel	3 mo	1000	December 2019
ATLANTIS[86] (Anti-Thrombotic Strategy After Trans-Aortic Valve Implantation for Aortic Stenosis) NCT02664649	Apixaban vs VKA or SAPT or DAPT	12 mo	1509	December 2019

dysfunction in 12,804 patients who had undergone TAVR, stratified according to the discharge antithrombotic treatment.[82] In this study, OAC (overwhelmingly with VKA), was independently associated with increased long-term mortality, despite adjustment for AF, emphasizing the need for a safer therapeutic alternative. It is important to realize that these data are nonrandomized and potentially subject to significant bias. Of note, VKA and NOACs have been associated in registry data and case reports with successful prevention and treatment of subclinical leaflet thrombosis compared with a single or dual antiplatelet strategy.[27]

It remains unclear whether patients who already have a baseline indication for OAC should receive additional antiplatelet therapy after TAVR. As per the European guidelines, a combination of VKA and lifelong aspirin is the current recommendation.[1] More recently, some nonrandomized, retrospective studies have noted potentially increased rates of major or life-threatening bleeding with the additional of antiplatelet agents to OACs, without a corresponding reduction in thromboembolic events.[83,84] One international registry comparing 621 patients showed that multiple antithrombotic therapies with a VKA + SAPT/DAPT versus VKA alone led to an increase in major or life-threatening bleeding (25.5% vs 14.9%, respectively; adjusted hazard ratio [HR] = 1.97, 95% CI, 1.11–3.51, P = .002) without differences in the composite of cardiovascular death, ischemic stroke, or myocardial infarction (16.4% vs 13.9%, respectively; adjusted HR = 1.33, 95% CI, 0.75–2.36, P = .33).[85]

Overall, ongoing randomized trials are warranted to clarify the net benefit of OAC in this high-risk group. The bleeding risk among these patients is generally high and the requirement for antiplatelet therapy is frequent given their inherent high atherothrombotic disease burden overlapping coronary disease with calcific AS. Most importantly, a bioprosthetic valve surface (and the related neo-sinus containing the disrupted native valve leaflets) is quite a different surface than the left atrium in patients with nonvalvular AF. Therefore, NOAC may not be appropriate at all.

ONGOING CLINICAL TRIALS

Several important clinical trials are currently ongoing, examining the question of antithrombotic therapy after TAVR.[86–88] These randomized trials are ongoing in intermediate-risk to high-risk patients; however, given the expected proliferation of TAVR into lower-risk populations in coming years, this topic will remain an ongoing investigation. These trials are examining antiplatelet and OAC in patients with and without indications for OAC at baseline. These studies can be categorized broadly according to whether there is a baseline indication for OAC or not, irrespective of the TAVR itself (Table 2).

SUMMARY

Balancing the potential bleeding, thrombotic, and ischemic complications after TAVR remains the greatest concern in the postprocedural period. Because of the high-risk profiles and frailty of this population, antithrombotic therapy after TAVR needs to be carefully evaluated. Furthermore, as TAVR RCTs continue to enroll lower-risk patients and challenge the paradigm of transcatheter therapies limited to higher risk populations, the risk of stroke and thromboembolic complications will become increasingly important.

There is equipoise between SAPT and DAPT for the prevention of thrombotic events after TAVR. There is no clear clinical benefit between OAC plus SAPT versus OAC alone in patients with an indication for chronic OAC. Bleeding is an important factor when deciding on a specific antithrombotic therapy, and this is a key clinical outcome in the RCTs that are evaluating the safety and efficacy of different post-TAVR pharmacologic strategies. Finally, OAC is useful for the treatment of bioprosthetic valve thrombosis, although this is a relatively rare clinical entity. In the opinions of the authors, SAPT or DAPT should be used after TAVR, based on other comorbidities and in the absence of an underlying indication for OAC. In the presence of underlying indication for OAC, OAC alone with possible addition of SAPT based on other comorbidities should be considered.

REFERENCES

1. Baumgartner H, Falk V, Bax JJ, et al. 2017 ESC/EACTS guidelines for the management of valvular heart disease. Eur Heart J 2017;38(36):2739–91.
2. Nishimura Rick A, Otto Catherine M, Bonow Robert O, et al. 2017 AHA/ACC focused update of the 2014 AHA/ACC guideline for the management of patients with valvular heart disease: a report of the American College of Cardiology/American Heart Association task force on clinical practice guidelines. Circulation 2017;135(25):e1159–95.

3. Mack MJ, Leon MB, Thourani VH, et al. Transcatheter aortic-valve replacement with a balloon-expandable valve in low-risk patients. N Engl J Med 2019;380(18):1695–705.

4. Popma JJ, Deeb GM, Yakubov SJ, et al, Evolut Low Risk Trial Investigators. Transcatheter aortic-valve replacement with a self-expanding valve in low-risk patients. N Engl J Med 2019;380(18):1706–15.

5. Cribier A. The development of transcatheter aortic valve replacement (TAVR). Glob Cardiol Sci Pract 2016;2016(4):e201632.

6. Dangas GD, Mehran R. Bleeding after aortic valve replacement matters: important mortality risk. JACC Cardiovasc Interv 2017;10(14):1447–8.

7. Genereux P, Cohen DJ, Mack M, et al. Incidence, predictors, and prognostic impact of late bleeding complications after transcatheter aortic valve replacement. J Am Coll Cardiol 2014;64(24):2605–15.

8. Holmes DR Jr, Mack MJ, Kaul S, et al. 2012 ACCF/AATS/SCAI/STS expert consensus document on transcatheter aortic valve replacement. J Am Coll Cardiol 2012;59(13):1200–54.

9. Webb J, Rodes-Cabau J, Fremes S, et al. Transcatheter aortic valve implantation: a Canadian Cardiovascular Society position statement. Can J Cardiol 2012;28(5):520–8.

10. Whitlock RP, Sun JC, Fremes SE, et al. Antithrombotic and thrombolytic therapy for valvular disease: antithrombotic therapy and prevention of thrombosis, 9th ed: American College of Chest Physicians evidence-based clinical practice guidelines. Chest 2012;141(2 Suppl):e576S–600S.

11. Ahmad Y, Demir O, Rajkumar C, et al. Optimal antiplatelet strategy after transcatheter aortic valve implantation: a meta-analysis. Open Heart 2018;5(1):e000748.

12. Leon MB, Smith CR, Mack MJ, et al. Transcatheter or surgical aortic-valve replacement in intermediate-risk patients. N Engl J Med 2016;374(17):1609–20.

13. Reardon MJ, Van Mieghem NM, Popma JJ, et al. Surgical or transcatheter aortic-valve replacement in intermediate-risk patients. N Engl J Med 2017;376(14):1321–31.

14. Smith CR, Leon MB, Mack MJ, et al. Transcatheter versus surgical aortic-valve replacement in high-risk patients. N Engl J Med 2011;364(23):2187–98.

15. Vranckx P, Valgimigli M, Windecker S, et al. Thrombo-embolic prevention after transcatheter aortic valve implantation. Eur Heart J 2017;38(45):3341–50.

16. Deviri E, Sareli P, Wisenbaugh T, et al. Obstruction of mechanical heart valve prostheses: clinical aspects and surgical management. J Am Coll Cardiol 1991;17(3):646–50.

17. Zoghbi WA, Chambers JB, Dumesnil JG, et al. Recommendations for evaluation of prosthetic valves with echocardiography and doppler ultrasound: a report from the American Society of Echocardiography's Guidelines and Standards Committee and the task force on prosthetic valves, developed in conjunction with the American College of Cardiology Cardiovascular Imaging Committee, Cardiac Imaging Committee of the American Heart Association, the European Association of Echocardiography, a registered branch of the European Society of Cardiology, the Japanese Society of Echocardiography and the Canadian Society of Echocardiography, Endorsed by the American College of Cardiology Foundation, American Heart Association, European Association of Echocardiography, a registered branch of the European Society of Cardiology, the Japanese Society of Echocardiography, and Canadian Society of Echocardiography. J Am Soc Echocardiogr 2009;22(9):975–1014.

18. Roudaut R, Serri K, Lafitte S. Thrombosis of prosthetic heart valves: diagnosis and therapeutic considerations. Heart 2007;93(1):137–42.

19. Mylotte D, Andalib A, Thériault-Lauzier P, et al. Transcatheter heart valve failure: a systematic review. J Am Coll Cardiol 2014;63(12 Suppl):A1727.

20. Hansson NC, Grove EL, Andersen HR, et al. Transcatheter aortic valve thrombosis: incidence, predisposing factors, and clinical implications. J Am Coll Cardiol 2016;68(19):2059–69.

21. Leetmaa T, Hansson Nicolaj C, Leipsic J, et al. Early aortic transcatheter heart valve thrombosis. Circ Cardiovasc Interv 2015;8(4):e001596.

22. Stortecky S, Windecker S. Stroke: an infrequent but devastating complication in cardiovascular interventions. Circulation 2012;126(25):2921–4.

23. Chen H, Power D, Giustino G. Optimal duration of dual antiplatelet therapy after PCI: integrating procedural complexity, bleeding risk and the acuteness of clinical presentation. Expert Rev Cardiovasc Ther 2018;16(10):735–48.

24. Dangas GD, Weitz JI, Giustino G, et al. Prosthetic heart valve thrombosis. J Am Coll Cardiol 2016;68(24):2670–89.

25. Puri R, Auffret V, Rodés-Cabau J. Bioprosthetic valve thrombosis. J Am Coll Cardiol 2017;69(17):2193–211.

26. Sorrentino S, Giustino G, Moalem K, et al. Antithrombotic treatment after transcatheter heart valves implant. Semin Thromb Hemost 2018;44(1):38–45.

27. Chakravarty T, Sondergaard L, Friedman J, et al. Subclinical leaflet thrombosis in surgical and transcatheter bioprosthetic aortic valves: an observational study. Lancet 2017;389(10087):2383–92.

28. Capodanno D, Petronio AS, Prendergast B, et al. Standardized definitions of structural deterioration and valve failure in assessing long-term durability of transcatheter and surgical aortic bioprosthetic valves: a consensus statement from the European Association of Percutaneous Cardiovascular Interventions (EAPCI) endorsed by the European Society of Cardiology (ESC) and the European Association for Cardio-Thoracic Surgery (EACTS). Eur J Cardiothorac Surg 2017;52(3):408–17.

29. Jilaihawi H, Asch FM, Manasse E, et al. Systematic CT methodology for the evaluation of subclinical leaflet thrombosis. JACC Cardiovasc Imaging 2017;10(4):461–70.

30. Makkar RR, Chakravarty T. Transcatheter aortic valve thrombosis: new problem, new insights. JACC Cardiovasc Interv 2017;10(7):698–700.

31. Pascual I, Carro A, Avanzas P, et al. Vascular approaches for transcatheter aortic valve implantation. J Thorac Dis 2017;9(Suppl 6):S478–87.

32. Piccolo R, Pilgrim T, Franzone A, et al. Frequency, timing, and impact of access-site and non-access-site bleeding on mortality among patients undergoing transcatheter aortic valve replacement. JACC Cardiovasc Interv 2017;10(14):1436–46.

33. Guedeney P, Mehran R, Collet JP, et al. Antithrombotic therapy after transcatheter aortic valve replacement. Circ Cardiovasc Interv 2019;12(1):e007411.

34. Guedeney P, Tchetche D, Petronio AS, et al. Impact of coronary artery disease and percutaneous coronary intervention in women undergoing transcatheter aortic valve replacement: from the WIN-TAVI registry. Catheter Cardiovasc Interv 2019;93(6):1124–31.

35. Gallo M, Putzu A, Conti M, et al. Embolic protection devices for transcatheter aortic valve replacement. Eur J Cardiothorac Surg 2018;53(6):1118–26.

36. Van Belle E, Hengstenberg C, Lefevre T, et al. Cerebral embolism during transcatheter aortic valve replacement: the BRAVO-3 MRI study. J Am Coll Cardiol 2016;68(6):589–99.

37. Kahlert P, Knipp SC, Schlamann M, et al. Silent and apparent cerebral ischemia after percutaneous transfemoral aortic valve implantation: a diffusion-weighted magnetic resonance imaging study. Circulation 2010;121(7):870–8.

38. Kahlert P, Al-Rashid F, Dottger P, et al. Cerebral embolization during transcatheter aortic valve implantation: a transcranial Doppler study. Circulation 2012;126(10):1245–55.

39. Van Mieghem NM, El Faquir N, Rahhab Z, et al. Incidence and predictors of debris embolizing to the brain during transcatheter aortic valve implantation. JACC Cardiovasc Interv 2015;8(5):718–24.

40. Schmidt T, Leon MB, Mehran R, et al. Debris heterogeneity across different valve types captured by a cerebral protection system during transcatheter aortic valve replacement. JACC Cardiovasc Interv 2018;11(13):1262–73.

41. Ghanem A, Kocurek J, Sinning JM, et al. Cognitive trajectory after transcatheter aortic valve implantation. Circ Cardiovasc Interv 2013;6(6):615–24.

42. Oldham MA, Vachon J, Yuh D, et al. Cognitive outcomes after heart valve surgery: a systematic review and meta-analysis. J Am Geriatr Soc 2018;66(12):2327–34.

43. Auffret V, Campelo-Parada F, Regueiro A, et al. Serial changes in cognitive function following transcatheter aortic valve replacement. J Am Coll Cardiol 2016;68(20):2129–41.

44. Nishimura RA, Otto CM, Bonow RO, et al. 2014 AHA/ACC guideline for the management of patients with valvular heart disease: a report of the American College of Cardiology/American Heart Association Task force on practice guidelines. J Thorac Cardiovasc Surg 2014;148(1):e1–132.

45. Jimenez Diaz VA, Tello-Montoliu A, Moreno R, et al. Assessment of platelet REACtivity after transcatheter aortic valve replacement: the REAC-TAVI trial. JACC Cardiovasc Interv 2019;12(1):22–32.

46. Riddle JM, Stein PD, Magilligan DJ, et al. Evaluation of platelet reactivity in patients with valvular heart disease. J Am Coll Cardiol 1983;1(6):1381–4.

47. Van Belle E, Rauch A, Vincent F, et al. Von Willebrand factor multimers during transcatheter aortic-valve replace. N Engl J Med 2016;375(4):335–44.

48. Polzin A, Schleicher M, Seidel H, et al. High on-treatment platelet reactivity in transcatheter aortic valve implantation patients. Eur J Pharmacol 2015;751:24–7.

49. Adams DH, Popma JJ, Reardon MJ, et al. Transcatheter aortic-valve replacement with a self-expanding prosthesis. N Engl J Med 2014;370(19):1790–8.

50. Durand E, Blanchard D, Chassaing S, et al. Comparison of two antiplatelet therapy strategies in patients undergoing transcatheter aortic valve implantation. Am J Cardiol 2014;113(2):355–60.

51. Koniari I, Kounis NG, Hahalis G. Antithrombotic treatment following transcatheter valve replacement: current considerations. J Thorac Dis 2017;9(11):4251–9.

52. Poliacikova P, Cockburn J, de Belder A, et al. Antiplatelet and antithrombotic treatment after transcatheter aortic valve implantation - comparison of regimes. J Invasive Cardiol 2013;25(10):544–8.

53. Sherwood MW, Vemulapalli S, Harrison JK, et al. Variation in post-TAVR antiplatelet therapy

utilization and associated outcomes: insights from the STS/ACC TVT Registry. Am Heart J 2018;204:9–16.

54. Rodes-Cabau J, Masson JB, Welsh RC, et al. Aspirin versus aspirin plus clopidogrel as antithrombotic treatment following transcatheter aortic valve replacement with a balloon-expandable valve: the ARTE (aspirin versus aspirin + clopidogrel following transcatheter aortic valve implantation) randomized clinical trial. JACC Cardiovasc Interv 2017;10(13):1357–65.

55. Stabile E, Pucciarelli A, Cota L, et al. SAT-TAVI (single antiplatelet therapy for TAVI) study: a pilot randomized study comparing double to single antiplatelet therapy for transcatheter aortic valve implantation. Int J Cardiol 2014;174(3):624–7.

56. Ussia GP, Scarabelli M, Mule M, et al. Dual antiplatelet therapy versus aspirin alone in patients undergoing transcatheter aortic valve implantation. Am J Cardiol 2011;108(12):1772–6.

57. Nijenhuis VJ, ten Berg JM, Hengstenberg C, et al. Usefulness of clopidogrel loading in patients who underwent transcatheter aortic valve implantation (from the BRAVO-3 randomized trial). Am J Cardiol 2019;123(9):1494–500.

58. Hu X, Yang FY, Wang Y, et al. Single versus dual antiplatelet therapy after transcatheter aortic valve implantation: a systematic review and meta-analysis. Cardiology 2018;141(1):52–65.

59. Hioki H, Watanabe Y, Kozuma K, et al. Pre-procedural dual antiplatelet therapy in patients undergoing transcatheter aortic valve implantation increases risk of bleeding. Heart 2017;103(5):361–7.

60. Zhao G, Zhou M, Ma C, et al. In-hospital outcomes of dual loading antiplatelet therapy in patients 75 years and older with acute coronary syndrome undergoing percutaneous coronary intervention: findings from the CCC-ACS (improving care for cardiovascular disease in China-acute coronary syndrome) project. J Am Heart Assoc 2018;7(7) [pii: e008100].

61. Fernandes Gilson C, Nasi G, Rivera M, et al. Abstract 18907: antithrombotic therapy after TAVR: an updated meta-analysis of single versus dual-antiplatelet therapy of randomized and propensity-matched studies. Circulation 2017;136(suppl_1):A18907.

62. Siddamsetti S, Balasubramanian S, Yandrapalli S, et al. Meta-analysis comparing dual antiplatelet therapy versus single antiplatelet therapy following transcatheter aortic valve implantation. Am J Cardiol 2018;122(8):1401–8.

63. Maes F, Stabile E, Ussia GP, et al. Meta-analysis comparing single versus dual antiplatelet therapy following transcatheter aortic valve implantation. Am J Cardiol 2018;122(2):310–5.

64. Makkar RR, Fontana G, Jilaihawi H, et al. Possible subclinical leaflet thrombosis in bioprosthetic aortic valves. N Engl J Med 2015;373(21):2015–24.

65. Yanagisawa R, Hayashida K, Yamada Y, et al. Incidence, predictors, and mid-term outcomes of possible leaflet thrombosis after TAVR. JACC Cardiovasc Imaging 2016. https://doi.org/10.1016/j.jcmg.2016.11.005.

66. Ruile P, Jander N, Blanke P, et al. Course of early subclinical leaflet thrombosis after transcatheter aortic valve implantation with or without oral anticoagulation. Clin Res Cardiol 2017;106(2):85–95.

67. Sondergaard L, De Backer O, Kofoed KF, et al. Natural history of subclinical leaflet thrombosis affecting motion in bioprosthetic aortic valves. Eur Heart J 2017;38(28):2201–7.

68. Levine GN, Bates ER, Bittl JA, et al. 2016 ACC/AHA guideline focused update on duration of dual antiplatelet therapy in patients with coronary artery disease. A report of the American College of Cardiology/American Heart Association task force on clinical practice guidelines. J Am Coll Cardiol 2016;68(10):1082–115.

69. Latib A, Naganuma T, Abdel-Wahab M, et al. Treatment and clinical outcomes of transcatheter heart valve thrombosis. Circ Cardiovasc Interv 2015;8(4) [pii:e001779].

70. Windecker S, Tijssen J, Giustino G, et al. Trial design: rivaroxaban for the prevention of major cardiovascular events after transcatheter aortic valve replacement: rationale and design of the GALILEO study. Am Heart J 2017;184:81–7.

71. Guedeney P, Chieffo A, Snyder C, et al. Impact of baseline atrial fibrillation on outcomes among women who underwent contemporary transcatheter aortic valve implantation (from the Win-TAVI Registry). Am J Cardiol 2018;122(11):1909–16.

72. Siontis GCM, Praz F, Lanz J, et al. New-onset arrhythmias following transcatheter aortic valve implantation: a systematic review and meta-analysis. Heart 2018;104(14):1208–15.

73. Tarantini G, Mojoli M, Urena M, et al. Atrial fibrillation in patients undergoing transcatheter aortic valve implantation: epidemiology, timing, predictors, and outcome. Eur Heart J 2017;38(17):1285–93.

74. Vora AN, Dai D, Matsuoka R, et al. Incidence, management, and associated clinical outcomes of new-onset atrial fibrillation following transcatheter aortic valve replacement: an analysis from the STS/ACC TVT registry. JACC Cardiovasc Interv 2018;11(17):1746–56.

75. Klomjit S, Vutthikraivit W, Thavaraputta S, et al. TCT-400 pre-existing atrial fibrillation increases mortality after transcatheter aortic valve

replacement: a meta-analysis. J Am Coll Cardiol 2017;70(18 Suppl):B164.

76. Jorgensen TH, Thygesen JB, Thyregod HG, et al. New-onset atrial fibrillation after surgical aortic valve replacement and transcatheter aortic valve implantation: a concise review. J Invasive Cardiol 2015;27(1):41–7.

77. Rashid HN, Gooley RP, Nerlekar N, et al. Bioprosthetic aortic valve leaflet thrombosis detected by multidetector computed tomography is associated with adverse cerebrovascular events: a meta-analysis of observational studies. EuroIntervention 2018;13(15):e1748–55.

78. Guedeney P, Vogel B, Mehran R. Non-vitamin K antagonist oral anticoagulant after acute coronary syndrome: is there a role? Interv Cardiol 2018; 13(2):93–8.

79. Ruff CT, Giugliano RP, Braunwald E, et al. Comparison of the efficacy and safety of new oral anticoagulants with warfarin in patients with atrial fibrillation: a meta-analysis of randomised trials. Lancet 2014;383(9921):955–62.

80. Seeger J, Gonska B, Rodewald C, et al. Apixaban in patients with atrial fibrillation after transfemoral aortic valve replacement. JACC Cardiovasc Interv 2017;10(1):66–74.

81. Seeger J, Gonska B, Rodewald C, et al. TCT-227 Apixaban in patients with atrial fibrillation after transfemoral aortic valve implantation compared with vitamin K antagonist. J Am Coll Cardiol 2016; 68(18 Suppl):B92.

82. Overtchouk P, Guedeney P, Rouanet S, et al. Long-term mortality and early valve dysfunction according to anticoagulation use: the FRANCE TAVI registry. J Am Coll Cardiol 2019;73(1): 13–21.

83. D'Ascenzo F, Benedetto U, Bianco M, et al. Which is the best antiaggregant or anticoagulant therapy after TAVI? A propensity-matched analysis from the ITER registry. The management of DAPT after TAVI. EuroIntervention 2017;13(12): e1392–400.

84. Geis NA, Kiriakou C, Chorianopoulos E, et al. Feasibility and safety of vitamin K antagonist monotherapy in atrial fibrillation patients undergoing transcatheter aortic valve implantation. EuroIntervention 2017;12(17):2058–66.

85. Abdul-Jawad Altisent O, Durand E, Munoz-Garcia AJ, et al. Warfarin and antiplatelet therapy versus warfarin alone for treating patients with atrial fibrillation undergoing transcatheter aortic valve replacement. JACC Cardiovasc Interv 2016;9(16): 1706–17.

86. Collet JP, Berti S, Cequier A, et al. Oral anti-Xa anticoagulation after trans-aortic valve implantation for aortic stenosis: the randomized ATLANTIS trial. Am Heart J 2018;200:44–50.

87. Nijenhuis VJ, Bennaghmouch N, Hassell M, et al. Rationale and design of POPular-TAVI: antiPlatelet therapy fOr Patients undergoing transcatheter aortic valve implantation. Am Heart J 2016;173:77–85.

88. Van Mieghem NM, Unverdorben M, Valgimigli M, et al. Edoxaban versus standard of care and their effects on clinical outcomes in patients having undergone transcatheter aortic valve implantation in atrial fibrillation-rationale and design of the ENVISAGE-TAVI AF trial. Am Heart J 2018;205: 63–9.

Bioprosthetic Valve Fracture for Valve-in-Valve Transcatheter Aortic Valve Replacement

Rationale, Patient Selection, Technique, and Outcomes

Mary Rodriguez Ziccardi, MD[a],
Elliott M. Groves, MD, MEng[b],*

KEYWORDS

- Bioprosthetic valve • Fracture • TAVR • Patient prosthesis mismatch • Valve in valve

---

KEY POINTS

- Patient–prosthesis mismatch is an issue that results in poor patient outcomes and typically affects those with a small annulus or those in whom an undersized valve is implanted.
- When a surgical bioprosthetic valve implant results in patient–prosthesis mismatch, the only option, until recently, was a repeat open procedure.
- Surgical valves are composed of multiple components, including a frame composed of a variety of materials. In some cases, this frame can be fractured with high-pressure balloon inflation.
- After fracture of a bioprosthetic valve, a transcatheter valve can be implanted and significantly increase the effective orifice area of the valve, thus reducing or in many cases eliminating patient–prosthesis mismatch.
- The technique for fracture, including the timing and type of valve implantation, must be carefully planned and executed to provide maximum benefit for the patient.

INTRODUCTION

Transcatheter aortic valve replacement (TAVR) is a safe and less invasive alternative to surgical aortic valve replacement (SAVR) for patients with severe aortic stenosis.[1–4] TAVR is a particularly excellent option for those patients with degeneration or malfunction of a previous surgical aortic valve bioprosthesis, because they are typically at intermediate-to-high risk of death with reoperation.[5,6] Placing a transcatheter valve inside a surgical bioprosthesis is referred to as valve-in-valve (ViV) TAVR, and has been approved by the United States Food and Drug Administration (FDA) for patients with failed surgical bioprosthetic valves in the aortic and mitral positions who have been evaluated by a multidisciplinary heart team.[5] Although ViV TAVR is becoming more frequent and is available in most experienced centers, significant limitations still exist. The size of the transcatheter valve implanted in TAVR is sized meticulously according to annular dimensions on preprocedural

---

Disclosures: None.
[a] Division of Cardiology, Department of Medicine, University of Illinois at Chicago, 840 South Wood Street Suite 920S, Chicago, IL 60612, USA; [b] Division of Cardiology, Department of Medicine, University of Illinois at Chicago, Jesse Brown VA Medical Center, 840 South Wood Street Suite 920S, Chicago, IL 60612, USA
* Corresponding author.
E-mail address: emgroves@uic.edu

Intervent Cardiol Clin 8 (2019) 373–382
https://doi.org/10.1016/j.iccl.2019.05.004

imaging; however, in ViV TAVR, the size of the transcatheter valve is limited by the inner diameter of the bioprosthetic valve in place. This limitation in transcatheter valve size, particularly in the setting of a small bioprosthesis, can lead to high postprocedure gradients, a phenomenon that is associated with poor clinical outcomes.[7] The Valve in Valve International (VIVID) registry found that high postprocedure gradients (>20 mm Hg) were more frequent in patients with a small (<21 mm) surgical valve prosthesis, and that those high gradients were associated with a high mortality risk within the first year after the procedure.[5] The cause of these inferior outcomes may be associated with a reduction in the effective orifice area (EOA) of the previously implanted surgical valve, inducing patient–prosthesis mismatch (PPM) if not present at baseline, or worsening PPM when present before TAVR.[8] Other than repeat surgical intervention, there was little recourse to correct PPM present after SAVR. However, the technique of bioprosthetic valve fracture (BVF) was developed to overcome high postprocedure gradients and PPM.

RATIONALE FOR BIOPROSTHETIC VALVE FRACTURE

The rationale for BVF involves the presence of PPM. PPM is a condition that is defined by a postprocedure EOA of an implanted prosthetic valve that is small in relation to patient body surface area (BSA). This mismatch produces a higher than expected transvalvular gradient compared with a normal-functioning prosthetic valve.[9–11] The physiopathology underlying the increased pressure gradient is a result of the accelerated transvalvular flow that is largely related to the stroke volume traveling through a small EOA.[12] Consistent with these physiologic considerations, the parameter to characterize PPM is the indexed EOA (EOAi), defined by the EOA of the prosthetic valve divided by the patient's BSA.[12] EOAi consistently correlates with the postprocedural gradients through a prosthetic valve.[13] The gradients increase exponentially when the indexed EOA ranges between 0.8 and 0.9 cm^2/m^2. Based on this, PPM is considered to be absent if the EOAi is greater than 0.85 cm^2/m^2, moderate if it is between 0.65 and 0.85 cm^2/m^2, and severe if less than 0.65 cm^2/m^2 (Box 1).[14] The severity of PPM is important and is directly associated with clinical outcomes.[13,14]

PPM concepts apply to all valves, but most of the literature has focused on the aortic valve. There are several reasons a patient can have

---

> **Box 1**
> **Grading criteria for patient prosthesis mismatch**
>
> - *Absent*: EOAi >0.85 cm^2/m^2
> - *Moderate*: EOAi >0.65 and ≤0.85 cm^2/m^2
> - *Severe*: EOAi <0.65 cm^2/m^2
>
> EOAi, indexed effective orifice area, defined as EOA divided by body surface area.

PPM. In the setting of surgical aortic valve replacement (SAVR), the 2 most important mechanisms are excessive annular calcification and a significant difference between the frame diameter and the inner diameter of the bioprosthesis.[14] Patients with aortic valve disease frequently have annular calcification and left ventricular hypertrophy, which reduce the size of the aortic annulus.[14] In severe cases, the annular calcium cannot be fully debulked during aortic valve replacement, and this in turn limits the size of the implanted prosthesis. The second reason mentioned relates to the valve itself. Depending on the type of prosthesis, the EOA can be significantly reduced by the anchoring or supporting system, the thickness of the leaflets, or the fabric cover, which is particularly relevant with stented valves.[14] **Fig. 1** demonstrates that the dimension of the valve is not the true inner diameter of the orifice, which is the only dimension relevant to the heart.

The prevalence of moderate PPM ranges between 20% and 70% depending on the study,

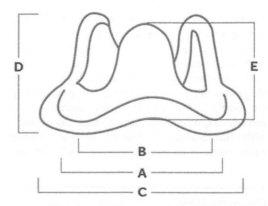

Fig. 1. The dimensions of a surgical aortic valve. A is the valve stent size, which is how the valve is labeled. However, B is the true inner diameter of the valve, which is what determines the effective orifice area. C is the outer diameter of the sewing ring. D is the valve height, and E is the aortic protrusion. In general, B is 1.5–3 mm less than A.

whereas that of severe PPM is between 2% and 11%.[15] In a meta-analysis of 58 studies that included a total of 40,381 patients who underwent SAVR or TAVR (39,568 and 813 patients, respectively), the overall incidence of PPM was 43.8%.[16] The incidence of PPM after TAVR is 36.7% according to the Society of Thoracic Surgery (STS)/American College of Cardiology (ACC) Transcatheter Valve Therapy (TVT) registry.[17] Of the 62,125 patients enrolled between 2014 and 2017 in the STS/ACC TVT registry, moderate and severe PPM was found in 12.1% and 24.6%, respectively.[17] In a meta-analysis of 108,182 patients treated with SAVR, the incidence of moderate/severe PPM was 53.7%.[18] In contrast, in the VIVID registry of patients with ViV TAVR, the incidence of any degree of PPM was 61%, with severe PPM in 24.6%.[19]

Several studies have shown that patient, anatomic, functional, valve, and procedure-related factors are predictors of the development of PPM.[16,17,20,21] Key patient factors include female sex, older age, clinical comorbidities, and patient size. Women often have smaller annuli, which increases the risk of a smaller EOA; furthermore, women tend to be older at the time of procedure, which is also an independent risk factor for PPM. Indeed, most studies have shown that older age is a strong predictive factor for PPM,[17,22] likely related to older patients receiving primarily bioprosthetic valves as opposed to mechanical valves, which increases the risk of PPM.[16,20] In contradistinction, in recent studies of patients mostly undergoing TAVR, younger age has been associated with PPM.[17,21–25] Clinical comorbidities that are related to the development of PPM include systemic hypertension, diabetes, and renal failure. Finally, a large BSA (PPM 1.85 m² versus no PPM 1.74 m², $P < .001$) and high body mass index (PPM 28.1 kg/m² versus no PPM: 25.9 kg/m², $P < .001$)[21] are associated with high rates of PPM.

Anatomic and functional factors that are associated with the development of PPM include a small aortic annular diameter; increased calcification of aortic annulus and aorta, which reduces the ability of the surgeon to implant an adequately sized valve; depressed left ventricular function; moderate to severe left ventricular hypertrophy; and increased left ventricular dimensions.

Valve- and procedure-related factors include valve size, valve type, and the procedure that is performed. A small valve prosthesis size (eg, ≤23 mm diameter) and a small baseline EOA and EOAi are associated with a greater risk of PPM.[17] Bioprosthetic valves have a 3-fold increased risk of PPM,[16] especially stented bioprosthetic valves. This might be secondary to the reduction of the EOA, with severe PPM secondary to the space occupied by the multiple components of the valve. Concomitant coronary artery bypass graft[16] and a ViV procedure are other procedure-related predictors.

EVALUATION FOR PATIENT–PROSTHESIS MISMATCH

PPM is first evaluated by a transthoracic echocardiogram (TTE). Typically, patients have increased gradients and velocities, consistent with aortic stenosis. If the valve leaflets are visible on TTE, they appear normal in cases of pure PPM. In addition, the acceleration time of the Doppler signal is less than 100 milliseconds.[13] However, in a patient with moderate PPM at baseline and concomitant degeneration, the leaflets may appear abnormal. To better visualize the leaflets, transesophageal echocardiography can be used. Finally, cardiac computed tomography (CT) gives a high-resolution image of the valve that can provide an assortment of adjunctive information. For example, CT can visualize leaflet thrombosis, which in the short-term after SAVR or TAVR can mimic PPM.[13] CT can also quantify the calcium burden on the leaflets; a higher calcium burden is associated with valvular stenosis and less likely with PPM. Finally, the CT scan determines sinus size; a significant valve to sinus size mismatch is suggestive of PPM. Ultimately, valves with PPM should be approached in a different manner when ViV TAVR is being considered, because simply implanting a new valve will not solve the issue and perhaps may exacerbate it.

PATIENT SELECTION FOR BIOPROSTHETIC VALVE FRACTURE

Patient selection for avoidance of PPM before any valve replacement is critical because of the significant impact on hemodynamics, functional recovery, and survival. Avoidance of the development of PPM can usually be accomplished by following a simple strategy at the time of operation that should be performed before each aortic valve replacement.[14,26] This approach was described by Pibarot and colleagues in a 3-step algorithm to prevent PPM[14]:

Step 1, calculate the BSA from patients' body weight and height; step 2, identify the minimum EOA of the prosthesis to be implanted to prevent PPM by multiplying the BSA by

$0.85 \text{ cm}^2/\text{m}^2$; step 3, choose the valve according to the results obtained and the reference values for the different types and sizes of valves.[27,28] If despite this assessment, PPM still projected, several options can be considered.[4] One can select a different type of valve with a bigger EOA such as a sutureless valve,[25] stentless bioprosthesis, mechanical or aortic homograft, or perform TAVR.[26] Alternatively, one can enlarge the aortic root to accommodate a larger prosthesis of the same type; this has been shown to reduce the incidence of PPM from 17% to 2.5% and without an increase in operative mortality risk.[27,28] With respect to TAVR, one can overexpand the selected transcatheter valve during the procedure and consider repositioning a self-expanding valve if an optimal position is not obtained initially.[21,23,28,29] Finally, in the case of a previous, failed bioprosthetic valve and the decision is to undergo ViV, fracturing the stent of the previous valve can be considered to reduce PPM.[17]

In low-risk patients, a more complex surgery involving a root enlargement generally does not add significant risk and can improve outcomes. However, in the low functional status/sedentary patient with a normal left ventricular ejection fraction, a moderate degree of PPM may be tolerable if there is an increased operative risk with modification of the aortic annulus or change of aortic valve replacement strategy due to selection of the valve.

When selecting a patient for BVF, several important considerations should be made. First, the patient should be evaluated fully for possible PPM. A patient with even mild PPM may progress to moderate PPM, and thus this must be taken into consideration. Generally, a small surgical valve is considered to be those with a labeled diameter of ≤21 mm, intermediate-sized valves are those with a labeled diameter of 22 to 25 mm, and larger valves are greater than 25 mm and are rarely affected by PPM. Small surgical valves should be considered for BVF, particularly if this would allow a larger transcatheter valve to be inserted. Although the data are somewhat limited, the data that are available suggest that a larger transcatheter valve with slight underexpansion will provide a lower postprocedure gradient than a fully expanded small valve in the same bioprosthetic annulus.[30] The temporal relationship between the patient's presentation and the index surgery must also be considered. If a patient is 15 years out from an SAVR and for 13 to 14 of those years was entirely asymptomatic, then it is unlikely that PPM is the driving force behind new symptoms, and

perhaps a high implant of a supra-annular valve would suffice and add no additional risk to the procedure. That being said, the initial experience with BVF has demonstrated a high degree of safety when proper planning is in place.

BIOPROSTHETIC VALVE FRACTURE TECHNIQUE

The dominant surgical strategy in aortic valve replacement is placement of a bioprosthetic valve. Surgical bioprosthetic valves are generally composed of a stent encompassed by a biocompatible fabric, a sewing ring, and leaflets composed of porcine or bovine pericardium. Surgical valve stents are composed of metallic (alloyed metal) and nonmetallic (polymer) materials that vary significantly in mechanical properties. For instance, the Mosaic Valve (Medtronic, Dublin, Ireland) has a sewing ring that is entirely nonmetallic, and the Magna and Magna Ease Valves (Edwards Lifesciences, Irvine, CA) have a sewing ring that is composed of a flexible cobalt-chromium alloy. As the stent provides the most significant contribution to the structural integrity of the valve, its composition must be understood.

As discussed previously, a significant proportion of surgical valves have some degree of PPM. Patients with PPM have worse outcomes, and the surgical bioprosthetic valves tend to degenerate at a higher rate than valves with an absence of PPM. Given the option of ViV TAVR, the degeneration of a surgical valve is no longer a catastrophic event that requires repeat surgery in a patient who is 10 to 20 years older than when they had their first sternotomy. However, ViV TAVR is not without limitations. By definition, the transcatheter valve must be placed inside the surgical valve; thus even if the surgical valve does not have some degree of PPM, a mismatch can be induced by placing a space-occupying object inside the valve.

Because of the challenges presented by ViV TAVR, a solution was required to overcome the issue of already present or induced PPM. Thus, BVF was developed on the benchtop and applied in a select patient population.[31] The technique is relatively simple but must be executed in a systematic manner and applied to the correct patient population. Fracturing the stent allows for a larger transcatheter valve to be implanted and mitigates the risk of PPM, which should provide the patient with better long-term outcomes.

Before the procedure, all imaging must be examined in great detail. The first dimensions to evaluate are the sinus diameters. If one is expanding a bioprosthetic valve, the sinus diameters must be large enough to accommodate the increased valve size without root rupture. Sinus diameters that are significantly larger than that of the valve also reduce the risk of coronary obstruction. Unlike routine TAVR, the most important consideration with ViV TAVR with regard to coronary obstruction is the distance from the coronary ostia to the final position of the bioprosthetic leaflets.[32] Generally, any leaflet to coronary ostia distance less than 3 mm is cause for concern. When BVF is performed, the gain in annular dimension is 3 to 4 mm, thus it has been suggested that at baseline, before BVF, the valve to coronary distance should be at least 5 mm to accommodate valve expansion.[32]

Surgical Valve Characteristics

To fracture a bioprosthetic valve stent, the composition of the stent must be amenable to fracture. For instance, valves with polymer stents such as the Epic (Abbott, Abbott Park, IL) and Mosaic are fractured relatively easily, whereas valves with a metal ring, such as the Trifecta (Abbott, Abbott Park, IL), cannot be fractured at any pressure. Finally, some metallic alloy rings, such as those in the Magna and Magna Ease, can be fractured at high pressures. The published data on the ability to fracture the various surgical valves are summarized in Table 1.[32]

How to Fracture

Fracturing a bioprosthetic valve is accomplished by way of high-pressure inflation of a balloon

Table 1
Published data on ability to fracture various surgical valves

Valve	Successful Fracture	Pressure (atm)
Abbott Trifecta	No	n/a
Abbott Biocor Epic	Yes	8
Medtronic Mosaic	Yes	10
Medtronic Handcock II	No	n/a
Sorin Mitroflow	Yes	12
Edwards Magna	Yes	24
Edwards Magna Ease	Yes	18

All pressures are with a TRUE balloon.
  Abbreviation: n/a, not available.
  Adapted from Allen KB, Chhatriwalla AK, Cohen DJ, et al. Bioprosthetic valve fracture to facilitate transcatheter valve-in-valve implantation. Ann Thorac Surg 2017;104:1501–8; with permission.

across the prosthetic valve annulus. In the usual fashion, a wire is placed across the valve into the left ventricle. The valvuloplasty balloon is placed across the prosthetic valve annulus. Typically, a balloon that is 1 mm larger than the valve stent diameter is chosen.[33] If the bioprosthetic valve is being fractured before the TAVR implant, it is preferable to place the balloon equally within the aorta and left ventricle. However, if the transcatheter valve has been implanted before fracture, then care must be taken to ensure that proper balloon sizing and placement is adhered to. If a CoreValve Evolut R or Pro (Medtronic, Dublin, Ireland) is implanted in a bioprosthetic valve before fracture, then several important considerations must be taken into account. The CoreValve family has several more dimensions than the balloon-expandable Sapien 3 and Sapien 3 Ultra valves (Edwards Lifesciences, Irvine, CA). These features, which are summarized in **Fig. 2**, include a waist diameter at the level of leaflet coaptation.[33] This waist diameter limits the balloon size that can be used. The balloon diameter cannot exceed the waist diameter by more than 2 mm without risking significant leaflet damage. In addition, the balloon should be placed significantly more ventricular when fracturing a valve after CoreValve placement to minimize the balloon crossing the waist and limit leaflet interaction. When a Sapien 3 or Sapien 3 Ultra has been placed, the use of an oversized balloon can again damage the leaflets; an oversized balloon can also dilate the stent to a point that leaflet coaptation is impaired, resulting in central regurgitation. This is in contrast to the CoreValve, which is a self-expanding nitinol stent with shape memory and will return to its intended size even if a larger balloon is used. For the Sapien, the maximal balloon diameter should not exceed the size of the valve by more than 2 mm. With a Sapien in place, the position of the balloon with regard to the ventricular and aortic components is less relevant because the Sapien valve is an annular valve, and the balloon will interact with the leaflets no matter where it is positioned.

Balloon choice is fairly limited given that the balloon must be rupture resistant and noncompliant with consistently accurate diameters. In practice and in the largest published case series, the balloons of choice are the TRUE valvuloplasty catheter and Atlas Gold percutaneous transluminal angioplasty (PTA) catheter (Bard, Franklin Lakes, NJ).[34] Both balloons are able to consistently fracture bioprosthetic valves with high-pressure inflations. The Atlas Gold is

	23 mm Evolut Pro/R	26 mm Evolut Pro/R	29 mm Evolut Pro/R	34 mm Evolut R
A. Inflow Diameter (mm)	23	26	29	34
B. Waist Diameter (mm)	20	22	23	24
C. Max Outflow Diameter (mm)	34	32	34	38
D. Commissure Height (mm)	26	26	26	26
E. Skirt Height (mm)	13	13	13	n/a
F. Frame Height (mm)	45	45	45	46

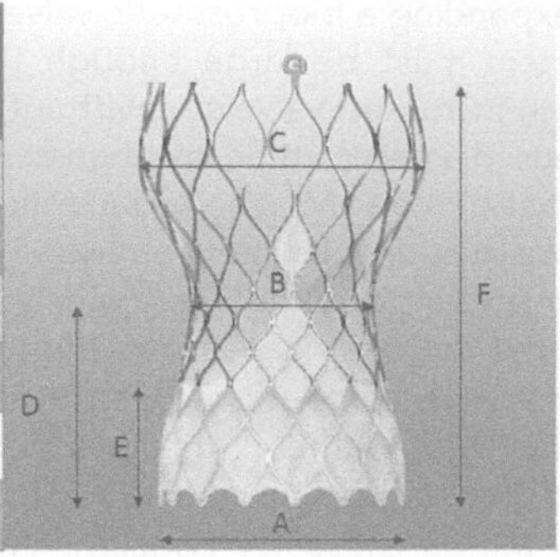

Fig. 2. This figure illustrates the dimensions of the CoreValve Evolut R and Pro. The dimension labeled by B, is the most important for BVF, because a balloon cannot be more than 2 mm larger than B without risking catastrophic valve damage. (*Reproduced with permission* of Medtronic, Inc.)

marketed as a PTA catheter and is less commonly stocked in structural heart labs, but is highly rupture resistant. The TRUE balloon is a noncompliant valvuloplasty balloon with a small diameter variance. As a result of its Kevlar coating and internal reinforcement, the balloon is highly rupture resistant and is ideal for the high-pressure inflations required for BVF.

Once the balloon is in the ideal position, the operator must be prepared for a high-pressure inflation. A hand inflation generally cannot reach a pressure of greater than 4 atm, whereas the easiest valves to fracture require at least 8 atm. Thus, some type of inflation device is necessary. However, inflating an 18 to 28 mm balloon with an inflation device is far too time consuming. Therefore, a 3-way stopcock is used, with a 60 mL syringe of diluted contrast to fill the balloon during a hand inflation placed on 1 port and an inflation device with sufficient volume to add several milliliters of volume is attached to the other (**Fig. 3**). Coronary inflation devices are commonly used, but they do present the risk of insufficient volume if the operator does not use the syringe properly. An alternative

is a large volume inflation device in addition to the syringe, for example, the Presto (Bard, Franklin Lakes, NJ) inflation device, which has a 30 mL chamber and can be inflated to 40 atm. Rapid pacing is started as the balloon is inflated as much as possible with the syringe; the stopcock is then turned to allow the balloon to reach high pressures using the inflation device.

Once the valve has been fractured, several signs are present (**Fig. 4**). The easiest to visualize and most reliable is the release of the balloon waist. Additional signs are a sudden decrease in pressure on the inflation device and an audible sound. Once the valve has been fractured, the balloon is deflated using the syringe and if necessary, the inflation device.

Valve Choice and Timing
An important decision to be considered is what type of transcatheter valve to implant and when to implant it, either before or after BVF. With regard to the timing of the implant, the operator must consider the risks and benefits of each approach. Fracturing the surgical valve before transcatheter valve implantation has several advantages but important disadvantages as well (**Table 2**). The most important benefit of fracture before implant is the avoidance of any potential damage to the transcatheter valve leaflets. However, the valve is universally crimped before implant, which can lead to tissue damage, and in the case of the supra-annular Core-Valve, the valvuloplasty balloon can be positioned in the annulus, but below the percutaneous valve leaflets. Another theoretic advantage is the ability to ensure that the bioprosthesis is fractured and thus implant a larger transcatheter valve. At this point in the experience with this procedure, successful fracture has been shown to be highly reproducible and thus a concern for lack of success should

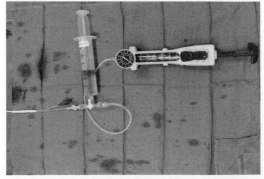

Fig. 3. A 3-way stopcock with a 60 mL syringe and high-pressure inflation device used to inflate a non-compliant balloon to high pressures.

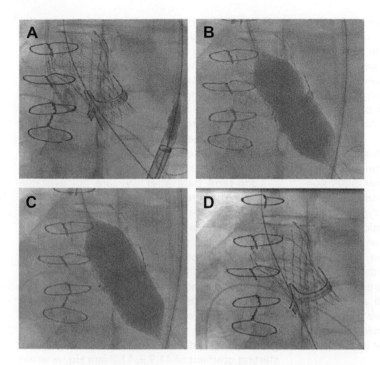

Fig. 4. (*A*) A significantly underexpanded CoreValve Evolut R has been implanted inside a Magna Valve. The valve appears underexpanded because it is oversized for the bioprosthesis. (*B*) A TRUE balloon is initially inflated and has a clear waist at the site of the neo annulus. (*C*) A uniform diameter of the balloon indicating that the valve has been fractured. (*D*) The fully expanded transcatheter valve with minimal residual gradient. (*Reproduced with permission* of Medtronic, Inc.)

not be a driving factor in decision making.[32] If the operators use a balloon-expandable transcatheter valve, then a fracture-first strategy may result in the need for a final high-pressure balloon inflation even after successful fracture.[32] This is because the delivery balloon used with the Sapien 3 is compliant and has been shown to be insufficient to fully expand the transcatheter valve. Thus, an additional high-pressure inflation is needed to fully expand the valve and realize the full hemodynamic benefits of the fracture strategy. This is less of an issue with a self-expanding valve, because the radial strength has been shown to be sufficient to realize the potential of maximal expansion after fracture and achieve maximal diameter. The most significant risk of a fracture-first strategy is acute severe aortic insufficiency, which can cause a patient to quickly deteriorate clinically. If this strategy is chosen, a valve should be fully ready for rapid deployment.

Fracture after implantation carries many benefits. First, the risk of acute decompensation and a hasty deployment is mitigated. In addition, there is evidence, albeit limited, that implantation of the percutaneous valve first provides a superior hemodynamic result. These data are confounded by significant differences in the type of valve implanted with significantly more balloon-expandable valve implantation after fracture without final high-pressure balloon inflation, and as was discussed earlier, this leads to suboptimal hemodynamics. Finally, there is no objective evidence that fracture after valve implantation leads to premature valve degeneration.

The type of valve chosen for ViV TAVR is generally dictated by several factors. Both the balloon-expandable Sapien 3/Sapien 3 Ultra and the self-expanding CoreValve Evolut Pro/R are excellent options and FDA approved for ViV TAVR. However, the case where the

Table 2			
Advantages and disadvantages of fracturing the surgical valve before and after transcatheter valve implantation			
BVF Before TAVR		**BVF After TAVR**	
Advantages	**Disadvantages**	**Advantages**	**Disadvantages**
Ensure successful BVF	Possible severe aortic	No risk of aortic	Possible BVF failure
Valve choice simple	insufficiency	insufficiency	Valve migration
	May need a second BAV	Better valve expansion	

operator is considering fracture typically involves bioprosthetic valves with a small annular dimension. This unique patient population has a significant amount of clinical data that generally, but not universally, support the use of a self-expanding valve.[28] This conclusion is primarily driven by the observations that in patients with a small annulus, the supra-annular CoreValve provides superior hemodynamics.[35] Specifically, in patients with a small annulus, the self-expanding valve was found to have a significantly lower peak velocity and higher dimensionless index. As mentioned previously, patients with moderate to severe PPM typically have valves with a small annular dimension, supporting the preference for a supra-annular valve. What must be considered, however, is that fracture of a bioprosthetic valve expands the annular diameter by 3 to 4 mm. That degree of annular expansion can easily shift a small annulus into the moderate range, whereby there is no statistically significant difference in dimensionless index between the supra-annular or intra-annular transcatheter valves.

The Mitral Position

The discussion so far has been directed toward the aortic position, but PPM can also occur in valves in the mitral position in some circumstances. Given the significantly higher volume of ViV TAVR compared with ViV transcatheter mitral valve replacement, there is less experience with BVF in the mitral position. However, there have been multiple case reports of success with mitral BVF.[36] The key consideration is the neo left ventricular outflow tract that is created. This would typically be a transseptal procedure, but otherwise, the same principles already discussed apply.

OUTCOMES AFTER BIOPROSTHETIC VALVE FRACTURE

The presence of PPM has been associated with worse outcomes after surgery.[12] Early mortality postprocedure is particularly important because the left ventricle is more vulnerable and sensitive to the increased hemodynamic burden imposed by PPM. This association is stronger when left ventricular dysfunction is present (67% mortality when left ventricular ejection fraction is <40%).[7] This may be related to underlying decreased ventricular reserve.[12] Long-term mortality is less dramatic, but still considerable, and the presence of an impact on late mortality might be related to accelerated valve degeneration that is associated with a baseline low

EOAi.[37,38] Less regression of left ventricular mass after aortic valve replacement has been described when PPM is present, and this is also associated with worse outcomes and higher mortality postprocedure.[4] Coronary hemodynamics, including a decrease in coronary flow reserve even in the absence of coronary artery disease, also likely play a role in the poor outcomes associated with PPM. This leads to a reduction in the symptomatic benefit derived by patients after SAVR or TAVR.[39,40]

Long-term data after BVF are not available because of the relative infancy of this technique. However, short-term data are encouraging. In a series of patients who underwent BVF to optimize hemodynamics, the mean gradient and EOA at 1 month postprocedure were statistically unchanged from the initial result, suggesting that the improvement in hemodynamics that is gained with BVF persists.[32] In a published series of the acute results, there was a striking lack of complications.[34] In this series, the mean postprocedure gradient was reduced to 6.7 ± 3.7 mm Hg from a starting gradient of 41.9 ± 11.2 mm Hg, whereas prefracture it was 20.5 ± 7.4 mm Hg. Given the available data on residual gradients greater than 20 mm Hg, this should be associated with improved long-term outcomes.

Durability concerns have been expressed after BVF given that the leaflets are subjected to high-pressure balloon inflation. This has been discussed earlier, and the converse point can be made that high residual gradients after ViV TAVR lead to accelerated valve degeneration and poor outcomes. Poorly expanded valves lead to premature failure given the change in maximal stress points that were not anticipated in the engineering process.[41] Procedural changes can also mitigate this issue with a more ventricular position of the balloon and the use of a supra-annular valve.

SUMMARY

SAVR is frequently complicated by PPM. PPM in turn leads to higher mortality and early valve degeneration. ViV TAVR has been an important tool in treating degenerated surgical valves, but is insufficient when treating PPM, and in fact, may worsen the situation. BVF may be performed to expand the annulus of the surgical valve and significantly improve hemodynamics after transcatheter valve placement. The technique is relatively simple and involves only small modifications to the standard balloon aortic valvuloplasty technique. Although short-term outcomes have been excellent, it remains to be seen if the subset of patients who undergo BVF have similar outcomes to those with low post-procedure gradients in the absence of BVF. Ultimately, BVF is a promising procedure that can be completed with a low rate of complications and provides the promise of improved long-term outcomes.

REFERENCES

1. Adams DH, Popma JJ, Reardon MJ. Transcatheter aortic valve replacement with a self-expanding prosthesis. N Engl J Med 2014;371:967–8.
2. Leon MB, Smith CR, Mack M, et al. Transcatheter aortic-valve implantation for aortic stenosis in patients who cannot undergo surgery. N Engl J Med 2010;363:1597–607.
3. Smith CR, Leon MB, Mack MJ, et al. Transcatheter versus surgical aortic-valve replacement in high-risk patients. N Engl J Med 2011;364:2187–98.
4. Leon MB, Smith CR. Transcatheter aortic-valve replacement. N Engl J Med 2016;375:700–1.
5. Dvir D, Webb JG, Bleiziffer S, et al. Transcatheter aortic valve implantation in failed bioprosthetic surgical valves. JAMA 2014;312:162–70.
6. Webb JG, Mack MJ, White JM, et al. Transcatheter aortic valve implantation within degenerated aortic surgical bioprostheses: PARTNER 2 valve-in-valve registry. J Am Coll Cardiol 2017;69:2253–62.
7. Blais C, Dumesnil JG, Baillot R, et al. Impact of prosthesis-patient mismatch on short-term mortality after aortic valve replacement. Circulation 2003;108:983–8.
8. Faerber G, Schleger S, Diab M, et al. Valve-in-valve transcatheter aortic valve implantation: the new playground for prosthesis-patient mismatch. J Interv Cardiol 2014;27:287–92.
9. Dumesnil JG, Honos GN, Lemieux M, et al. Validation and applications of indexed aortic prosthetic valve areas calculated by Doppler echocardiography. J Am Coll Cardiol 1990;16:637–43.
10. Dumesnil JG, Honos GN, Lemieux M, et al. Validation and applications of mitral prosthetic valvular areas calculated by Doppler echocardiography. Am J Cardiol 1990;65:1443–8.
11. Dumesnil JG, Yoganathan AP. Valve prosthesis hemodynamics and the problem of high transprosthetic pressure gradients. Eur J Cardiothorac Surg 1992;6(suppl):S34–7.
12. Pibarot P, Dumesnil JG. Prosthesis-patient mismatch: definition, clinical impact, and prevention. Heart 2006;92(8):1022–9.
13. Zoghbi WA, Chambers JB, Dumesnil JG, et al. Recommendations for evaluation of prosthetic valves with echocardiography and Doppler ultrasound: a report from the American Society of Echocardiography's Guidelines and Standards Committee and the Task Force on Prosthetic Valves, developed in conjunction with the American College of Cardiology Cardiovascular Imaging Committee, Cardiac Imaging Committee of the American Heart Association, the European Association of Echocardiography, a registered branch of the European Society of Cardiology, the Japanese Society of Echocardiography and the Canadian Society of Echocardiography. J Am Soc Echocardiogr 2009;22:975–1014.
14. Pibarot P, Dumesnil JG. Hemodynamic and clinical impact of prosthesis-patient mismatch in the aortic valve position and its prevention. J Am Coll Cardiol 2000;36:1131–41.
15. Pibarot P, Dumesnil JG. Prosthetic heart valves: selection of the optimal prosthesis and long-term management. Circulation 2009;119:1034–48.
16. Dayan V, Vignolo G, Soca G, et al. Predictors and outcomes of prosthesis-patient mismatch after aortic valve replacement. JACC Cardiovasc Imaging 2016;9:924–33.
17. Herrmann HC, Daneshvar SA, Fonarow GC, et al. Prosthesis-patient mismatch in patients undergoing transcatheter aortic valve replacement: from the STS/ACC TVT registry. J Am Coll Cardiol 2018;72:2701.
18. Sa MPBO, de Carvalho MMB, Sobral Filho DC, et al. Surgical aortica valve replacement and patient prosthesis mismatch: a meta-analysis of 108 182 patients. Eur J Cardiothorac Surg 2019. https://doi.org/10.1093/ejcts/ezy466.
19. Bleiziffer S, Erlebach M, Simonato M, et al. Incidence, predictors and clinical outcomes of residual stenosis after aortic valve-in-valve. Heart 2018;104:828–34.
20. Bonderman D, Graf A, Kammerlander AA, et al. Factors determining patient-prosthesis mismatch after aortic valve replacement—a prospective cohort study. PLoS One 2013;8:e81940.
21. Liao Y-B, Li Y-J, Jun-Li L, et al. Incidence, predictors and outcome of prosthesis-patient mismatch after transcatheter aortic valve replacement: a systematic review and meta-analysis. Sci Rep 2017;7:15014.
22. Fallon JM, DeSimone JP, Brennan JM, et al. The incidence and consequence of prosthesis-patient mismatch after surgical aortic valve replacement. Ann Thorac Surg 2018;106:14–22.
23. Pibarot P, Weissman NJ, Stewart WJ, et al. Incidence and sequelae of prosthesis-patient mismatch in transcatheter versus surgical valve replacement in high-risk patients with severe aortic stenosis: a PARTNER trial cohort-A analysis. J Am Coll Cardiol 2014;64:1323–34.
24. Thyregod HG, Steinbrüchel DA, Ihlemann N, et al. No clinical effect of prosthesis-patient mismatch after transcatheter versus surgical aortic valve replacement in intermediate- and low risk patients with severe aortic valve stenosis at mid-term

follow-up: an analysis from the NOTION trial. Eur J Cardiothorac Surg 2016;50:721–8.

25. Tully PJ, Aty W, Rice GD, et al. Aortic valve prosthesis patient mismatch and long-term outcomes: 19- year single-center experience. Ann Thorac Surg 2013;96:844–50.

26. Pibarot P, Dumesnil JG, Cartier PC, et al. Patient-prosthesis mismatch can be predicted at the time of operation. Ann Thorac Surg 2001;71:S265–8.

27. Lancellotti P, Pibarot P, Chambers J, et al. Recommendations for the imaging assessment of prosthetic heart valves: a report from the European Association of Cardiovascular Imaging endorsed by the Chinese Society of Echocardiography, the Interamerican Society of Echocardiography and the Brazilian Department of Cardiovascular Imaging. Eur Heart J Cardiovasc Imaging 2016;17:589–90.

28. Hahn RT, Leipsic J, Douglas PS, et al. Comprehensive echocardiographic assessment of normal transcatheter valve function. JACC Cardiovasc Imaging 2019;12:25–34.

29. Bavaria JE, Desai ND, Cheung A, et al. The St Jude Medical Trifecta aortic pericardial valve: results from a global, multicenter, prospective clinical study. J Thorac Cardiovasc Surg 2014;147:590–7.

30. Azadani AN, Reardon M, Simonato M, et al. Effect of transcatheter aortic valve size and position on valve-in-valve hemodynamics: an in vitro study. J Thorac Cardiovasc Surg 2017;153:1303–15.

31. Tanase D, Grohmann J, Schubert S, et al. Cracking the ring of Edwards Perimount bioprosthesis with ultrahigh pressure balloons prior to transcatheter valve in valve implantation. Int J Cardiol 2014;176:1048–9.

32. Saxon JT, Allen KB, Cohen DJ, et al. Bioprosthetic valve fracture during valve-in-valve TAVR: bench to bedside. Interv Cardiol 2018;13(1):20–6.

33. Yudi MB, Sharma SK, Tang GHL, et al. Coronary angiography and percutaneous coronary intervention after transcatheter aortic valve replacement. J Am Coll Cardiol 2018;71:1360–78.

34. Chhatriwalla AK, Allen KB, Saxon JT, et al. Bioprosthetic valve fracture improves the hemodynamic results of valve-in-valve transcatheter aortic valve replacement. Circ Cardiovasc Interv 2017;10:e005216.

35. Rogers T, Steinvil A, Gai JT, et al. Choice of balloon-expandable versus self-expanding transcatheter aortic valve impacts hemodynamics differently according to aortic annular size. Am J Cardiol 2017;119:900–4.

36. Kamioka N, Corrigan F, Iturbe JM, et al. Mitral bioprosthetic valve fracture: bailout procedure for undersized bioprosthesis during mitral valve-in-valve procedure with paravalvular leak closure. JACC Cardiovasc Interv 2018;11:e21–2.

37. Tasca G, Mhagna Z, Perotti S, et al. Impact of prosthesis-patient mismatch on cardiac events and mortality after aortic valve replacement in patients with pure aortic stenosis. Circulation 2006;113:570–6.

38. Nardi P, Russo M, Saitto G, et al. The prognostic significance of patient-prosthesis mismatch after aortic valve replacement. Korean J Thorac Cardiovasc Surg 2018;51(3):161–6.

39. Gould KL, Carabello BA. Why angina in aortic stenosis with normal coronary arteriograms? Circulation 2003;107:3121–3.

40. Marcus ML, Doty DB, Hiratzka LF, et al. Decreased coronary reserve: a mechanism for angina pectoris in patients with aortic stenosis and normal coronary arteries. N Engl J Med 1982;307:1362–6.

41. Abbasi M, Azadani AN. Leaflet stress and strain distributions following incomplete transcatheter aortic valve expansion. J Biomech 2015;48:3663–71.

Percutaneous Approaches to the Treatment of Mitral Leaflet Perforation and to Residual Regurgitation After Transcatheter Edge-to-Edge Mitral Valve Repair

Marvin H. Eng, MD[a],*, Tiberio M. Frisoli, MD[b],
Adam B. Greenbaum, MD[c], Pedro Villablanca, MD[b],
Dee Dee Wang, MD[b], James Lee, MD[b],
William O'Neill, MD[b]

KEYWORDS

- Mitral valve leaflet perforation • Occluder device • Mitral regurgitation
- Transcatheter mitral valve repair

KEY POINTS

- Despite the clinical success of transcatheter edge-to-edge mitral valve repair, residual postprocedural mitral regurgitation can occur between MitraClips or at the commissures, which can be challenging to address.
- Mitral valve leaflet perforation can result in severe mitral regurgitation and cannot be addressed with transcatheter edge-to-edge repair; percutaneous implantation of an occluder device may be considered in patients at high or prohibitive risk for open surgery and who are not anatomic candidates for enrollment in clinical trials of transcatheter mitral valve replacement.
- The technical approach for percutaneous occluder implantation for mitral regurgitation includes retrograde wiring of the mitral valve lesion from the left ventricular outflow tract, snaring of the guidewire within the left atrium, and occluder delivery through an anterograde from the femoral vein.
- Percutaneous implantation of the CARDIOFORM Septal Occluder requires premature removal of the retrieval cord so that the atrial disc forms correctly after deployment.
- Complications of occluder placement within mitral valve lesions include device embolization, residual regurgitation, and hemolysis; the latter may be a particular issue with nitinol weave-based devices.

 Video content accompanies this article at http://www.interventional.theclinics.com.

Conflicts of interest: Dr M.H. Eng is a clinical proctor for Edwards Lifesciences. Drs T.M. Frisoli, J. Lee, and P. Villablanca have no conflicts to declare. Dr D.D. Wang is a consultant to Boston Scientific, Edwards Lifesciences, and Materialise. Dr W. O'Neill is a consultant to Abiomed, Medtronic, and Boston Scientific. Dr A.B. Greenbaum is a proctor for Edwards Lifesciences, Medtronic, and Abbott Vascular; holds equity in and has been a scientific advisor for Transmural Systems; and has received institutional research support from Edwards Lifesciences, Abbott Vascular, Medtronic, and Boston Scientific.

[a] Center for Structural Heart Disease, Henry Ford Hospital, 2799 West Grand Boulevard, Detroit, MI 48202, USA;
[b] Henry Ford Hospital, 2799 West Grand Boulevard, Detroit, MI 48202, USA; [c] Emory University Hospital, 550 Peachtree Street Northeast, Fl 6, Suite 600, Atlanta, GA 30308, USA
* Corresponding author. Center for Structural Heart Disease, Henry Ford Hospital, Clara Ford Pavilion 434, 2799 West Grand Boulevard, Detroit, MI 48236.
E-mail address: Meng1@hfhs.org

Intervent Cardiol Clin 8 (2019) 383–391
https://doi.org/10.1016/j.iccl.2019.06.001
2211-7458/19/© 2019 Elsevier Inc. All rights reserved.

INTRODUCTION

Mitral valve disease is prevalent in 9% to 10% of patients $\geq$75 years old, a growing population globally.[1] Although surgery remains the gold standard, it is precarious in elderly patients because the 30-day mortality has been reported to be as high as 11% and 18.9% for repair and replacement, respectively.[2] As a result, many patients are left untreated: only 15% of patients from a US population study were referred for surgery.[3] Therefore, innovative transcatheter mitral valve therapies have been developed to treat the aging population, resulting in multiple devices for both repair and valve replacement.[4,5] As the field of interventional cardiology expands, more unique scenarios will emerge whereby clinicians may encounter challenging situations that cannot easily be addressed using established repair or replacement technologies. In this article, the authors reflect on their experience with the percutaneous repair of leaflet perforations and failed edge-to-edge mitral valve procedures.[6]

BASIC ANATOMY OF THE MITRAL VALVE LEAFLETS

Selecting the best approach for mitral valve repair or replacement centers on individualized patient anatomy. The mitral valve is composed of 2 leaflets, the annular attachment at the atrioventricular junction, tendinous cords, and papillary muscles (**Fig. 1**). The 2 leaflets are most commonly described as anterior and posterior.[7] The anterior leaflet accounts for one-third of the annular circumference and shares a fibrous continuity with the left and noncoronary cusps of the aortic valve as well as the interleaflet triangle between the coronary cusps abutting the membranous septum.[7,8] This proximity to the aortic valve is particularly important; the opening of the anterior leaflet in diastole nears the left ventricular outflow tract (LVOT). Carpentier's model describes the most lateral segment as A1, the central segment as A2, and the medial segment as A3.[9] The posterior leaflet accounts for the remaining two-thirds of the left atrioventricular junction and is usually not as broad as the anterior leaflet. The posterior leaflet has indentations that form 3 scallops along the line of coaptation. To mirror the designation of the anterior leaflet, the most lateral segment of the posterior leaflet is referred to as P1, the central as P2, and the most medial as P3.

The anatomic mechanism of mitral regurgitation has commonly been classified using Carpentier's system for describing mitral valve pathologic condition relative to the mitral annular plane. Type 1 describes the case of normal leaflet motion, with the mitral regurgitation a result of causes, such as leaflet perforation or annular dilation from atrial fibrillation. Type 2 describes excessive leaflet motion above the annular plane, most commonly from leaflet prolapse. In type 3, there is leaflet restriction; this category is further divided into 2 subtypes. In type 3a, there is restriction of leaflet motion in both systole and diastole (ie, rheumatic disease), whereas in 3b, there is restriction in systole only (ie, ischemic heart disease or dilated cardiomyopathy).[9]

Multiple devices are under development for repairing the mitral valve that focus on different anatomic and functional components: leaflet, annulus, and chordal attachment. The most mature technology addresses the valve leaflets using the concept of edge-to-edge repair, first described as the surgical Alfieri stitch technique.[10] The MitraClip (Abbott Vascular, Santa Clara, CA, USA) and the PASCAL device (Edwards Lifesciences, Irvine, CA, USA) both aim to capture isolated segments of the anterior and posterior leaflets and permanently bind them together to reduce regurgitation. The degree of reduction in mitral regurgitation is the strongest predictor of long-term survival after intervention: a multicenter German registry found procedure failure to be associated with a 4.36-fold increase in 1-year mortality.[11] Residual mitral regurgitation remains a clinical dilemma for clinicians given that candidates for percutaneous mitral valve repair are either poor or prohibitive candidates for surgery and the percutaneous approach is usually the last remaining option.

Mitral valve replacement seems to be a logical alternative to the prospects of an inadequate repair. Transcatheter mitral valve replacement (TMVR) remains investigational in the United States, and a number of potential candidates is currently vying for commercial approval.[12] However, in the short experience with TMVR, some limitations in generalizing the procedure to a larger population have been noted. For instance, many valves are delivered transapically, and historical experience with surgical transapical access during the transcatheter aortic valve replacement experience was associated with high mortalities without symptomatic benefit.[13] Furthermore, the wide variability in patient anatomy causes significant challenges resulting in high screen-fail rates during investigational mitral valve studies.[14] Not only is annular fit a challenge but also the proximity to the LVOT has prompted concerns of

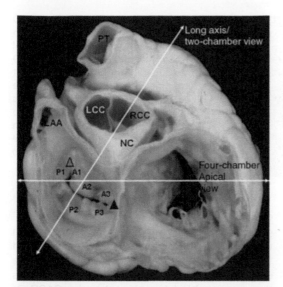

Fig. 1. Mitral valve anatomy from the perspective of the left atrium. The anterolateral commissure (Δ) is adjacent to the left atrial appendage (LAA), and the line of coaptation extends in a curved line toward the interatrial septum, ending at the posteromedial commissure (▲). The anterior leaflet (A1-A3) abuts the aortic valve, whereas the posterior leaflet (P1-3) attaches to the posterior myocardium. Using the Carpentier system, the most lateral is termed "1," and most medial segments of each leaflet is "3." LAA, left atrial appendage; LCC, left coronary cusp; NC, non-coronary cusp; RCC, right coronary cusp. (Adapted from McCarthy, K.P., L. Ring, and B.S. Rana, Anatomy of the mitral valve: understanding the mitral valve complex in mitral regurgitation. Eur J Echocardiogr, 2010. 11(10): p. i3-9; with permission.)

displacing the anterior leaflet into the LVOT causing obstruction during systole.[15] Another factor that limits the generalizability of TMVR is the need for oral anticoagulation after implantation.[16,17] Several observational studies have noted the proclivity for thrombus formation, possibly because of remaining native leaflets creating pockets of stasis near the prosthetic valve and a milieu for thrombosis.[17,18] Although the cause has yet to be confirmed, oral anticoagulation appears to be required early after all TMVR cases, and the optimal duration of thromboprophylaxis remains unclear. Given these challenges, TMVR may not apply to every given patient, and therefore, repair may be the preferable approach.

There are certain leaflet anatomies that are not suitable for edge-to-edge repair, such as isolated leaflet perforations, leaflet tears, or residual regurgitation between MitraClips. To address these unique scenarios, clinicians have creatively used several occluder devices in an off-label fashion to treat perforations or failed

percutaneous repairs in a manner similar to treating perivalvular mitral valve leaks (Box 1).

CASE EXAMPLE: TREATMENT OF RESIDUAL LEAK BETWEEN MitraClips

An 88-year-old woman who had previously undergone edge-to-edge valve repair developed significant residual mitral valve regurgitation causing New York Heart Association (NYHA) class III symptoms. Two years before, the patient underwent transcatheter edge-to-edge repair using 3 MitraClips. She subsequently developed residual regurgitation between 2 MitraClips, and there was insufficient space to insert another clip. Because she was deemed to be at prohibitive risk for surgery by the heart team, the authors proceeded to try transcatheter placement of an occluder in an attempt to reduce the severity of mitral regurgitation. Under 3-dimensional transesophageal echocardiographic (TEE) guidance, the authors achieved transseptal access using an SL-1 catheter (Abbott Vascular) and BRK-1 XS transseptal needle (Abbott Vascular), then exchanging for a medium curl Agilis catheter (Abbott Vascular). Subsequently, the defect was crossed using a straight stiff glide wire (Terumo, Somerset, NJ, USA) to exchange for an extra-small curl Safari wire (Medtronic, St. Paul, MN, USA) via a 5-F pigtail catheter. Over the Safari wire, a 6-F 45° Torque View catheter (Abbott Vascular) tracked into the left ventricle (LV) to deliver a 9-mm Amplatzer muscular ventricular septal defect (VSD) occluder. Another 6/6-mm Amplatzer Duct Occluder (ADO) II (Abbott Vascular) was deployed with little reduction in mitral regurgitation (Fig. 2). In the following days, transfusion-dependent hemolytic anemia developed, and her heart failure symptoms persisted. A second attempt at inserting an ADO II next to the VSD occluder and obliterating any remaining regurgitation did not successfully reduce mitral

---

Box 1
Occluder devices previously used for percutaneous mitral repair

Amplatzer Duct Occluder II (Abbott Vascular, Santa, Clara, CA, USA)

Amplatzer Vascular Plug II (Abbott Vascular)

Amplatzer Septal Occluder (Abbott Vascular)

Amplatzer Vascular Plug III (Abbott Vascular)

CARDIOFORM Septal Occluder (GORE, Flagstaff, AZ, USA)

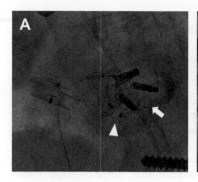
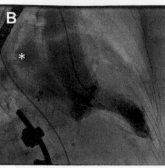

Fig. 2. Placement of VSD and ADO II devices between MitraClips in an attempt to treat residual mitral regurgitation. (*A*) A 9-mm VSD occluder (*arrowhead*) is placed at the medial edge of the clips, while a 6/6 ADO II occluder (*arrow*) is deployed between 2 of the clips. (*B*) Left ventriculogram demonstrating moderate to severe mitral regurgitation (*asterisk*) despite occluder placement.

regurgitation, and the patient subsequently expired because of respiratory failure.

CASE EXAMPLE: OCCLUSION OF MITRAL LEAFLET PERFORATION WITH AN AMPLATZER CRIBIFORM OCCLUDER

A 61-year-old woman with severe mitral regurgitation, end-stage renal disease, and lower-extremity amputation presented with a focal perforation near the base of the anterior leaflet at the A2 location[6] (Fig. 3). She was deemed at prohibitive surgical evaluation risk, and therefore, percutaneous repair was attempted. The authors' strategy consisted of grasping the leaflet using a MitraClip, retrogradely crossing the defect at the base of the leaflet, building an arterial-venous rail, and then deploying an occluder device. Concern for compromising leaflet coaptation from the occluder device prompted the strategy of using a MitraClip to stabilize the mitral valve. The authors grasped the leaflets at A2-P2 near the perforation and closed the clip very slowly, careful to watch the defect and to make sure closing the clip did enlarge it. After plicating the A2-P2 segments, the authors advanced a 6-Fr intramuscular (IM) guide into the LV and directed a glidewire into the left atrium through the leaflet perforation in a retrograde fashion from the LVOT. After deploying the MitraClip, the authors exchanged the MitraClip guide catheter for a medium curl Agilis steerable catheter (Abbott Vascular) to snare and externalize the glidewire, thereby creating an arterial-venous loop. The authors first delivered a 5-F Torque View LP catheter (Abbott Vascular) and deployed an ADO II, but the device embolized into the left atrium while still attached to the delivery cable. Next, the arterial-venous loop was reestablished, and a CARDIOFORM Septal Occluder was used. In order to deliver the occluder device, the CARDIOFORM delivery system was disassembled to separate the catheter and the CARDIOFORM

device. A dilator from a 7-F Torque View 45° guide (Abbott Vascular) was inserted through the CARDIOFORM delivery catheter and used to advance the delivery catheter across the defect. The CARDIOFORM delivery system was then reassembled by reinserting the CARDIOFORM occluder device into the delivery catheter while underwater to ensure no air was introduced to the LV. The CARDIOFORM was deployed in standard fashion with the distal disc in the LV and the proximal disc in the left atrium. Although the occluder sealed the defect, deployment of the CARDIOFORM device in the standard fashion resulted in the retrieval cord tensioning the proximal disc and not allowing it to form appropriately (see Fig. 3). The authors were concerned that this would create a nidus for thrombus, and therefore, the device was recaptured, and they then implanted an 18-mm Amplatzer Cribiform Septal Occluder (Abbott Vascular). Mitral regurgitation was reduced to mild, but hemolytic anemia ensued. After intermittent blood transfusions for 3 months, the hemolysis relented. The patient's dyspnea improved to NYHA functional class II requiring no further interventions.

CASE EXAMPLE: OCCLUSION OF MITRAL PERFORATION WITH A CARDIOFORM SEPTAL OCCLUDER

A 66-year-old man with a history of nonalcoholic steatohepatitis and severe mitral regurgitation owing to an A1 perforation presented with heart failure.[6] Referred for percutaneous repair, the procedural steps from the perforation described above were recapitulated. However, this time the CARDIOFORM was released "backwards," where the retrieval cord was first withdrawn so that no tension would present on the proximal disc (Fig. 4, Online Videos 1 and 2). At this point, if recapture was required, snaring would be necessary. The authors then uncoupled the catheter from the device, and without the retrieval

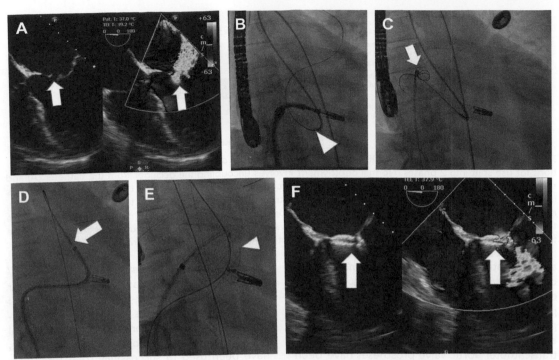

Fig. 3. Process of creating an arterial-venous loop to treat an anterior mitral leaflet perforation. Attempt at occluding the defect was unsuccessful using a 15-mm CARDIOFORM device; however, subsequent placement of an 18-mm Cribiform device did reduce mitral regurgitation, but hemolysis followed. (A) Severe mitral regurgitation through a circumscribed perforation near the base of the anterior mitral valve leaflet (arrows). (B) MitraClip deployment and retrograde crossing of the anterior leaflet perforation with a 6-F IM guide catheter and soft angled glidewire (arrowhead). (C) Agilis catheter and Atrieve snare capture the glidewire to externalize out the venous access (arrow). (D) Delivery of the CARDIOFORM delivery catheter coupled with a 7-F dilator through the leaflet perforation into the LVOT (arrow). (E) Deployment of the CARDIOFORM Occluder under tension from the retrieval cord deformed the proximal disc (arrowhead). (F) Implantation of an 18-mm Amplatz Cribiform Occluder (arrow) with stable positioning and mild residual mitral regurgitation.

cord, the proximal disc properly formed its intended shape, sealing the perforation and reducing the mitral regurgitation to trivial (Fig. 5). Postprocedure and 1-year echocardiogram demonstrated a stable device with trivial mitral regurgitation.

CASE EXAMPLE: TREATMENT OF FAILED TRANSCATHETER MITRAL VALVE REPAIR WITH THE CARDIOFORM SEPTAL OCCLUDER

A 77-year-old man with severe chronic obstructive pulmonary disease and a prolonged hospitalization was found to have severe degenerative mitral regurgitation. While undergoing MitraClip implantation, 1 clip was deployed, but attempts to treat a residual lateral jet of regurgitation resulted in posterior leaflet tear, and further attempts to place a clip were unsuccessful. The procedure was stopped, and the authors resolved to attempt percutaneous

exclusion of the lateral mitral orifice using a CARDIOFORM contingent on an acceptable mitral valve gradient. Once transseptal access was achieved, the authors directed a J-tipped wire into the LV using a medium-curve Agilis, enabling exchange for a pigtail catheter and subsequently a stiff wire. A 30-mm CARDIOFORM Septal Occluder was deployed "backwards" and initially the mitral regurgitation improved to mild. Unfortunately, follow-up echocardiography demonstrated an embolized device with recurrent severe mitral regurgitation (Fig. 6). Ultimately, the patient succumbed to drug-resistant pneumonia and died 2 weeks later.

MITRAL LEAFLET PERFORATION

Mitral perforation is a relatively infrequent finding, but it has been reported several times in the literature, arising from a variety of causes, including endocarditis, iatrogenic, autoimmune,

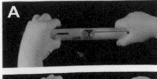
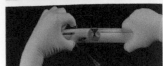
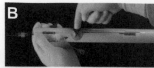
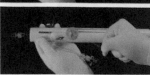

Fig. 4. Deployment steps for the GORE CARDIOFORM Occluder device according to the manufacturer instructions for use split into 2 phases. Normal deployment involves uncoupling the occluder from the catheter (A) and then removing the retrieval cord, which completely detaches the occluder device from the deployment apparatus (B). When deploying the GORE CARDIOFORM in the mitral position, the retrieval cord tensions the proximal disc, not allowing it to take its natural "flat" conformation. Proper formation of the proximal disc can be achieved if the tension is completely removed by pulling out the retrieval cord first (B) and then uncoupling the occluder device from the catheter (A). (*Courtesy of* W.L. Gore & Associates, Inc, Flagstaff, AZ; with permission.)

and idiopathic.[19–25] Perforations from endocarditis are relatively rare with 1 high-volume single center reporting 26 perforations over a 19-year period.[21] Several cases of late anterior leaflet perforation occurring from interactions with either balloon-expandable or self-expanding transcatheter aortic valve prostheses have been published.[20,26] Cardiac surgery, pacemaker implantation, radiofrequency ablation, and even Impella insertion have been implicated in mitral leaflet perforation, suggesting that as clinicians continue to expand the breadth of care, iatrogenic leaflet injuries will continue.

RESIDUAL MITRAL REGURGITATION AFTER TRANSCATHETER EDGE-TO-EDGE REPAIR

Residual mitral regurgitation after edge-to-edge repair is not infrequent. Data from the EVEREST (EndoVascular valve Edge-to-edge REpair Study) -II trial demonstrated a 21% rate of 3 to 4+ post–clip mitral regurgitation, although operator experience has subsequently improved, as a 7% rate of 3 to 4+ post–clip mitral regurgitation was

observed in the US Society of Thoracic Surgery/ American College of Cardiology Transcatheter Valve Therapy registry.[27,28] When the source of residual regurgitation is between clips, treatment is particularly problematic if surgical replacement is not an option. ADO II devices have been used to successfully treat regurgitation between clips.[29] Although the authors' attempt to use VSD and ADO II devices to treat mitral regurgitation was unsuccessful, it demonstrated that devices can be placed between clips, and perhaps appropriately sized expanded polytetrafluoroethylene (ePTFE) -based devices could treat these lesions more successfully and reduce the risk of hemolysis.

Deployment of the CARDIOFORM Septal Occluder in the mitral space is unique for several reasons. The delivery catheter is designed to treat septal defects and does not have an obturator or tapered shape. It is delivered in a rapid exchange fashion, and therefore, the edge of catheter orifice can snag soft tissue and potentially disrupt delicate structures and therefore requires operators to disassemble the delivery system

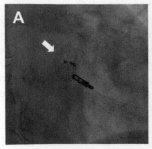
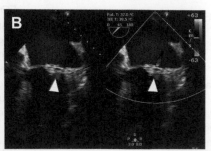

Fig. 5. Implantation of a 25-mm GORE CARDIOFORM "backwards" but pulling the retrieval cord first and then uncoupling the occluder from the catheter. (A) The CARDIOFORM distal and proximal discs (*arrow*) have taken their natural conformation because it was deployed without any tension in contrast to the appearance in **Fig. 3**E. (B) TEE images of the CARDIOFORM (*arrowhead*) again with trivial residual mitral regurgitation. (*Courtesy of* W.L. Gore & Associates, Inc, Flagstaff, AZ; with permission.)

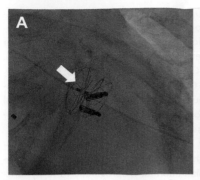 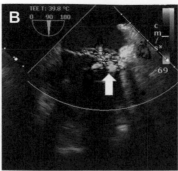 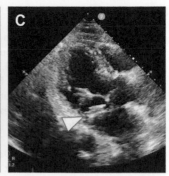

Fig. 6. Implantation of a 30-mm CARDIOFORM to seal a leaflet tear caused by a MitraClip transcatheter mitral valve repair device. (*A*) Attempts to place a second MitraClip caused a posterior leaflet tear, and the patient declined the surgery, prompting placement of the CARDIOFORM (*arrow*) to address the residual mitral regurgitation. (*B*) Initial placement of the device decreased residual mitral regurgitation to mild (*arrow*). (*C*) Transthoracic echocardiogram 24 hours postoccluder implantation revealed an embolized device (*arrowhead*). (*Courtesy of* W.L. Gore & Associates, Inc, Flagstaff, AZ.)

separating the delivery catheter from the CARDIOFORM occluder device, using a dilator from a 7-F system to couple to delivery catheter and reassemble the delivery system inside the body. In addition, because the catheter is relatively straight, shaping the catheter with a heat gun is performed to improve deliverability when treating mitral valves. The third unique facet of using the CARDIOFORM device in the mitral position is removing tension from the retrieval cord to allow the proximal disc to form appropriately. Therefore, if operators want to use the CARDIOFORM Occluder to repair mitral defects, they must accept not being able to recapture the device after locking, because the tension must be released from the system by releasing the retrieval cord before it is uncoupled from the catheter.[6]

Material such as ePTFE appears to be a favorable material for occluding defects. It is soft and conformable, and there should be less concern for hemolysis compared with woven nitinol occluders. Thus far, the authors' experience with woven nitinol devices at the mitral valve has shown occasional hemolysis, consistent with other reports in the literature.[6,23] Because leaflet erosion could occur when nitinol devices are placed adjacent to the mitral valve for left atrial appendage occlusion and perivalvular leak repair, placing them within or next to the mitral leaflets for treatment of leaflet perforation or residual mitral regurgitation after edge-to-edge repairs raises concern over long-term safety as well.[30,31] Given the concerns over possible hemolysis and erosion, perhaps softer devices composed of fabric may be more suited for this clinical situation.

All of the authors' cases used MitraClip to stabilize the leaflet before deploying occluder devices within the mitral valve. The authors'

theoretic concerns were that without the stability of the clip, the added weight to the leaflet could disrupt coaptation. However, several cases have been reported where nitinol devices were deployed without incident and no MitraClip was used.[23,32] Therefore, in the future, these cases will likely be attempted without prior edge-to-edge repair; however, publication bias and sparse data make generalizations challenging.

SUMMARY

In summary, use of occluder devices in percutaneous mitral leaflet repair is feasible, but the caveats of hemolysis and embolization remain. There is a larger experience with nitinol-based devices; however, the CARDIOFORM Septal Occluder shows promise. Its use does require unconventional deployment to properly form both discs; otherwise, the proximal disc will be malformed if deployed under tension. The literature is populated by case reports only, and long-term efficacy and safety of the devices for this application are not known. Rigorous clinical workup and anatomic analysis confirming the absence of active endocarditis, sufficient tissue to stabilize an occluder device, and technical expertise in mitral perivalvular leak repair are fundamental aspects needed for success. Proliferation of cardiovascular procedures will likely lead to more obscure complications, such as leaflet injury and residual regurgitation, between edge-to-edge repair devices requiring tertiary centers to meet this challenge.

SUPPLEMENTARY DATA

Supplementary data related to this article can be found online at https://doi.org/10.1016/j.iccl. 2019.06.001.

REFERENCES

1. Nkomo VT, Gardin JM, Skelton TN, et al. Burden of valvular heart diseases: a population-based study. Lancet 2006;368(9540):1005–11.

2. Chikwe J, Goldstone AB, Passage J, et al. A propensity score-adjusted retrospective comparison of early and mid-term results of mitral valve repair versus replacement in octogenarians. Eur Heart J 2011;32(5):618–26.

3. Dziadzko V, Clavel MA, Dziadzko M, et al. Outcome and undertreatment of mitral regurgitation: a community cohort study. Lancet 2018; 391(10124):960–9.

4. Regueiro A, Granada JF, Dagenais F, et al. Transcatheter mitral valve replacement: insights from early clinical experience and future challenges. J Am Coll Cardiol 2017;69(17):2175–92.

5. Maisano F, Alfieri O, Banai S, et al. The future of transcatheter mitral valve interventions: competitive or complementary role of repair vs. replacement? Eur Heart J 2015;36(26):1651–9.

6. Frisoli TM, Greenbaum A, O'Neill WW, et al. Percutaneous repair of mitral valve leaflet perforation. JACC Cardiovasc Interv 2019;12(2):210–3.

7. Ho SY. Anatomy of the mitral valve. Heart 2002; 88(suppl 4):iv5–10.

8. Ormiston JA, Shah PM, Tei C, et al. Size and motion of the mitral valve annulus in man. I. A two-dimensional echocardiographic method and findings in normal subjects. Circulation 1981;64(1): 113–20.

9. Filsoufi F, Carpentier A. Principle in reconstructive surgery in degenerative mitral valve disease. Semin Thorac Cardiovasc Surg 2007;19:103–10.

10. Alfieri O, Maisano F, De Bonis M, et al. The double orifice technique in mitral valve repair: a simple solution for complex problems. J Thorac Cardiovasc Surg 2001;122:674–81.

11. Puls M, Lubos E, Boekstegers P, et al. One-year outcomes and predictors of mortality after Mitra-Clip therapy in contemporary clinical practice: results from the German transcatheter mitral valve interventions registry. Eur Heart J 2016;37(8): 703–12.

12. Preston-Maher GL, Torii R, Burriesci G. A technical review of minimally invasive mitral valve replacements. Cardiovasc Eng Technol 2015;6(2):174–84.

13. Blackstone EH, Suri RM, Rajeswaran J, et al. Propensity-matched comparisons of clinical outcomes after transapical or transfemoral transcatheter aortic valve replacement: a placement of aortic transcatheter valves (PARTNER)-I trial substudy. Circulation 2015;131(22):1989–2000.

14. Bapat V, Rajagopal V, Meduri C, et al. Early experience with new transcatheter mitral valve replacement. J Am Coll Cardiol 2018;71(1):12–21.

15. Wang DD, Eng MH, Greenbaum AB, et al. Validating a prediction modeling tool for left ventricular outflow tract (LVOT) obstruction after transcatheter mitral valve replacement (TMVR). Catheter Cardiovasc Interv 2017;92(2):379–87.

16. Eng MH, Greenbaum A, Wang DD, et al. Thrombotic valvular dysfunction with transcatheter mitral interventions for postsurgical failures. Catheter Cardiovasc Interv 2017;90(2):321–8.

17. Cheung A, Webb JG, Barbanti M, et al. 5-year experience with transcatheter transapical mitral valve-in-valve implantation for bioprosthetic valve dysfunction. J Am Coll Cardiol 2013;61(17):1759–66.

18. Heras M, Chesebro JH, Fuster V, et al. High risk of thromboemboli early after bioprosthetic cardiac valve replacement. J Am Coll Cardiol 1995;25(5): 1111–9.

19. Ari H, Kahraman F, Arslan A, et al. Late perforation of anterior mitral leaflet after surgical resection of the subaortic membrane. J Cardiol Cases 2015; 12(6):199–201.

20. Amat-Santos IJ, Cortes C, Varela-Falcon LH. Delayed left anterior mitral leaflet perforation and infective endocarditis after transapical aortic valve implantation—case report and systematic review. Catheter Cardiovasc Interv 2017;89(5):951–4.

21. Sareyyupoglu B, Schaff HV, Suri RM, et al. Safety and durability of mitral valve repair for anterior leaflet perforation. J Thorac Cardiovasc Surg 2010;139(6):1488–93.

22. Mashicharan M, Cowburn PJ, Livesey SA, et al. Anterior mitral valve perforation in the absence of acute infection: diagnosis by two-dimensional and three-dimensional transesophageal echocardiography. Echocardiography 2017;34(12):1953–5.

23. Velasco S, Larman M, Eneriz M. Percutaneous closure of a native mitral valve perforation. Rev Esp Cardiol 2010;63(5):597.

24. Eftekhari A, Eiskjær H, Terkelsen CJ, et al. Perforation of the anterior mitral leaflet after Impella LP 5.0 therapy in cardiogenic shock. Am J Cardiol 2016; 117(9):1539–41.

25. Han J, Xu J, He Y. Anterior mitral leaflet perforation: a rare complication of radiofrequency ablation for paroxysmal supraventricular tachycardia. Clin Case Rep 2017;5(8):1414–5.

26. Saji M, Ailawadi G, Ragosta M, et al. Anterior mitral leaflet perforation during transcatheter aortic valve replacement in a patient with mitral annular calcification. JACC Cardiovasc Interv 2015;8(13):e215–6.

27. Feldman T, Foster E, Glower DD, et al. Percutaneous repair or surgery for mitral regurgitation. N Engl J Med 2011;364(15):1395–406.

28. Sorajja P, Vemulapalli S, Feldman T, et al. Outcomes with transcatheter mitral valve repair in the United States: an STS/ACC TVT registry report. J Am Coll Cardiol 2017;70(19):2315–27.

29. Kubo S, Cox JM, Mizutani Y, et al. Transcatheter procedure for residual mitral regurgitation after mitraclip implantation using Amplatzer Duct Occluder II. JACC Cardiovasc Interv 2016;9(12): 1280–8.

30. Rogers JH, Morris AS, Takeda PA, et al. Bioprosthetic leaflet erosion after percutaneous mitral paravalvular leak closure. JACC Cardiovasc Interv 2010;3(1):122–3.

31. Berrebi A, Sebag FA, Diakov C, et al. Early anterior mitral valve leaflet mechanical erosion following left atrial appendage occluder implantation. JACC Cardiovasc Interv 2017;10(16):1708–9.

32. Klapyta A, Pręgowski J, Chmielak Z, et al. Bail-out use of the Amplatzer Septal Occluder for treatment of acute iatrogenic leaflet perforation during the MitraClip procedure in a patient with functional mitral regurgitation. Postepy Kardiol Interwencyjnej 2018;14(3):304–8.

Transcatheter Aortic Valve Replacement with the Lotus Valve
Concept and Current State of the Data

Lennart van Gils, MD, PhD, Nicolas M. Van Mieghem, MD, PhD*

KEYWORDS

- Lotus valve • Mechanically expanded valve • Aortic stenosis
- Transcatheter aortic valve replacement

KEY POINTS

- Transcatheter aortic valve replacement (TAVR) with the mechanically expanded Lotus valve is intuitive and forms a valuable adjunct to the range of transcatheter heart valve (THV) platforms.
- Current data confirm excellent long-term clinical outcomes (ie, mortality and stroke) after TAVR with the Lotus valve in higher surgical risk populations compared with self-expanding and balloon-expandable THVs, and results in intermediate-risk patients are awaited.
- Hemodynamic performance of the Lotus valve is characterized by slightly smaller effective orifice area than supra-annular designs but is eminently suited for eliminating paravalvular leak.
- Conduction disturbances represent the Lotus valve's Achilles heel, although new device iterations and sizing algorithms may help mitigate this issue.

INTRODUCTION

Transcatheter aortic valve replacement (TAVR) has become the standard treatment of patients with severe aortic stenosis and increased surgical risk.[1,2] Recently, TAVR with Sapien 3 (Edwards Lifesciences, Irvine, CA) and Evolut R/Pro (Medtronic, Minneapolis, MN) have also been shown to be noninferior for major clinical outcomes (ie, death, stroke, rehospitalization) compared with surgery in low-risk patients.[3,4] Conduction disorders and residual paravalvular leaks (PVLs) remain prevalent and may have even more clinical weight in young low-risk patients. Several new transcatheter heart valve (THV) concepts have entered the market and currently provide an interesting range of THV options for the treatment of severe aortic stenosis. In the current era, operators should select the THV that is optimal for each individual patient. The Lotus THV (Boston Scientific, Marlborough, MA) is the only mechanically expanded platform, and this article discusses its device characteristics and clinical outcomes.

THE CONCEPT

The Lotus valve system consists of a trileaflet bovine pericardial valve supported by a braided nitinol frame (**Fig. 1**). A central radiopaque marker facilitates THV positioning within the aortic root. The frame is covered with an adaptive seal at the inflow segment that conforms to aortic root irregularities and mitigates PVL.

The Lotus valves are available in 3 sizes (23, 25, and 27 mm) covering a range of annulus diameters from 19 to 27 mm. They are either delivered through an 18-Fr sheath (23-mm valve) or a 20-Fr sheath (25-mm and 27-mm valves).

Department of Interventional Cardiology, Thoraxcenter, ErasmusMC, Room Rg-628, 's Gravendijkwal 230, Rotterdam 3015 CE, The Netherlands
* Corresponding author.
E-mail address: n.vanmieghem@erasmusmc.nl

Intervent Cardiol Clin 8 (2019) 393–402
https://doi.org/10.1016/j.iccl.2019.06.002
2211-7458/19/© 2019 Elsevier Inc. All rights reserved.

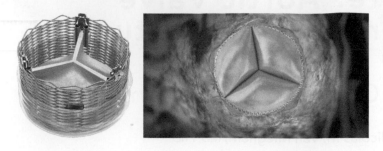

Three buckles at the top of the frame are connected to the delivery system through 3 coupling fingers. The nitinol frame expands on unsheathing. The unique feature of Lotus is the subsequent locking mechanism, which approximates the buckles (top of the frame) with the posts (level of valve leaflets), comparable with fastening a seatbelt. The frame shortens from the top down from a height of 70 mm to 19 mm during the locking process (**Fig. 2**). After locking, the valve is fully deployed and functional, but at this stage the valve can still be repositioned or even completely retrieved. At this juncture, the position relative to the coronary ostia and presence of paravalvular aortic regurgitation can be assessed. This option to either retrieve or reposition the valve after complete deployment and before release is a unique and crucial feature of the Lotus technology.

The delivery system has an ergonomic and intuitive handle. Rotating the blue control knob counterclockwise unsheathes and locks the THV, and clockwise rotation results in resheathing. Ultimately, the release cover proximal to

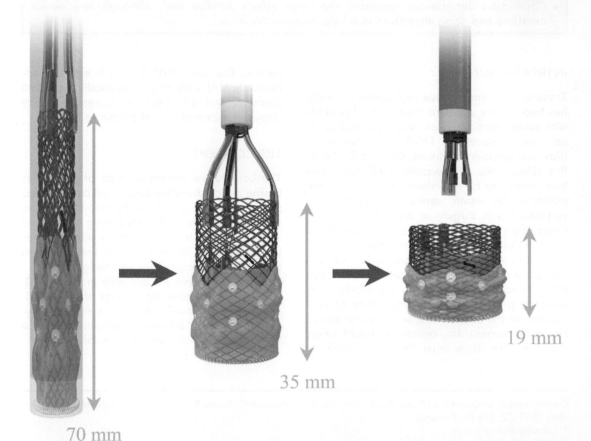

Fig. 2. The process of foreshortening during the different implantation steps: fully sheathed (*left*); fully unsheathed (*middle*); locked and released (*right*). (©2019 Boston Scientific Corporation or its affiliates. All rights reserved.)

the blue control knob can be slid forward to release the valve from the catheter.

Fig. 3 shows the implantation technique step by step. The implantation involves 3 separate steps: unsheathing, locking, and releasing.

CLINICAL DATA REVIEW
Long-term Survival Outcome
The larger Lotus trials reported consistent outcomes in terms of survival. The Repositionable Percutaneous Replacement of Stenotic Aortic Valve Through Implantation of Lotus Valve (REPRISE) II trial enrolled 120 patients with a mean Society of Thoracic Surgeons (STS) score of 7.1% and reported an all-cause mortality of 10.9%.[5] These favorable outcomes with Lotus were confirmed within the REPRISE-III and the Re-positionable Lotus Valve System – Post Market Evaluation of Real World Clinical Outcomes (RESPOND) studies.

REPRISE-III was a randomized controlled trial of 912 patients treated with Lotus or CoreValve in a 2:1 ratio, with mean STS scores of 6.7%

and 6.9%, respectively.[6] Lotus showed a similar survival outcome compared with CoreValve (all-cause mortality, 11.9% vs 13.5%, respectively). The recently published 2-year outcomes of this trial continue to report similar survival, with a 21.3% all-cause mortality with Lotus versus 22.5% with CoreValve.[7] The RESPOND postmarket registry analyzed a real-world population of 996 patients with a mean STS score of 6.0%[8]; all-cause mortality at 1 year was 11.7%.

One-year survival rates after TAVR with the Lotus valve within REPRISE-III and RESPOND are comparable with equally sized trials with different THV platforms in patients with similar risk profiles. Fig. 4 shows all-cause mortalities across the large TAVR trials. In the US Core-Valve High Risk Study (mean STS score, 7.3%), TAVR with CoreValve was associated with lower rates of mortality compared with surgical aortic valve replacement (SAVR) at 1-year follow-up (14.2% vs 19.1%, respectively),[9] and this benefit remained at 2-year follow-up

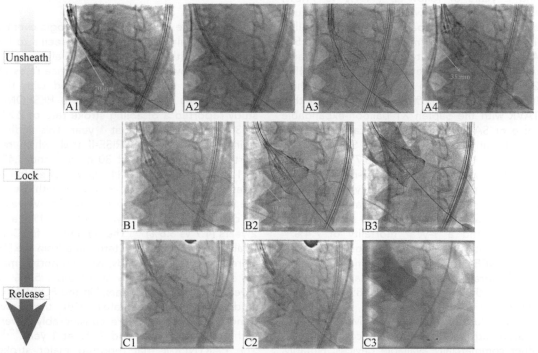

Fig. 3. Fluoroscopic views of the stepwise implantation process. Unsheathing: (A1) fully sheathed Lotus valve (frame height, 70 mm) with the distal tip of the nitinol frame below the native annulus; (A2, A3) unsheathing of the valve. The valve functions early during deployment; (A4) fully unsheathed valve (frame height, 35 mm). Locking: (B1) locking of the frame in a correct fluoroscopic image with all buckles and posts visible; (B2) fully locked frame (frame height shrinks to 19 mm); (B3) angiogram to confirm correct Lotus position after locking and assess paravalvular regurgitation. At this stage, the valve is still fully repositionable and can be resheathed. Release: (C1, C2) disconnecting the fingers from the frame buckles; (C3) final angiogram to evaluate position and paravalvular regurgitation. (©2019 Boston Scientific Corporation or its affiliates. All rights reserved.)

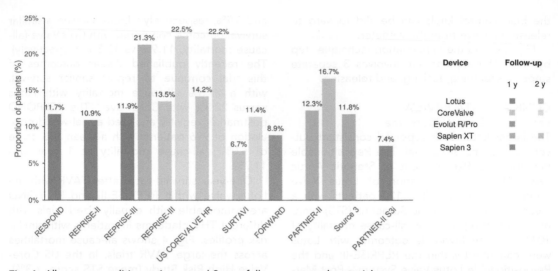

Fig. 4. All-cause mortalities at 1-year and 2-year follow-up across large trials.

(22.2% vs 28.6%, respectively).[10] In the Surgical Replacement and Transcatheter Aortic Valve Implantation (SURTAVI) trial, TAVR was associated with similar survival outcome compared with SAVR at 1 year (6.7% vs 6.8%, respectively) and 2 years of follow-up (11.4% vs 11.6%, respectively).[11] The Evolut R FORWARD study evaluated the self-expanding Evolut R enrolled 1040 patients with a mean STS score of 5.5%. At 1-year, the mortality was 8.9%.[12] The Placement of Aortic Transcatheter Valves (PARTNER) 2A trial compared an intermediate-risk cohort (mean STS score, 5.8%) who underwent either TAVR with the Sapien XT balloon-expandable valve or SAVR.[13] Reported all-cause mortality was similar between TAVR and SAVR (1 year, 12.3% vs 12.9%; 2 years, 16.7% vs 18.0%, respectively). A large propensity-matched analysis from the Sapien 3 observational study investigated 1077 patients treated with the Sapien 3 valve with a mean STS score of 5.2% and reported a 1-year mortality of 7.4%.[14] In the multicenter Source 3 registry (Logistic EuroSCORE 14%), all-cause mortality after transfemoral TAVR with the Sapien 3 valve was slightly higher with 11.8% at 1-year follow-up.[15]

In conclusion, long-term survival in patients treated with the Lotus valve is consistent with other commercially available devices. Notably, both REPRISE-III and RESPOND trials investigated a patient population that was at higher estimated surgical risk compared with other intermediate-risk trials and registries. At present, there are no longer-term clinical outcome data available for Lotus in intermediate-risk patients. The single-arm Lotus Edge Valve System

in Intermediate Surgical Risk Subjects (REPRISE IV) trial (ClinicalTrials.gov identifier: NCT03618095) will enroll 896 intermediate-risk patients (STS score between 3.0 and 8.0) and is currently recruiting.

Stroke

In general, the incidence of neurologic events, and in particular disabling stroke, seems to be acceptable with use of the Lotus valve. **Fig. 5** provides an overview of the incidence rates of major stroke with Lotus compared with the other devices in larger trials. The RESPOND study reported a disabling stroke rate of 2.2% at 30 days,[16] and 4.1% at 1 year. This finding is in line with the REPRISE-II trial, which reported a rate of 1.7% at 30 days,[17] and 3.4% at 1 year.[5] The REPRISE-III study showed lower rates of disabling stroke associated with use of the Lotus valve compared with the CoreValve at 30 days (2.0 vs 3.3%), 1 year (3.6 vs 7.1%), and 2 years (4.7 vs 8.6%).[6,7] These numbers for CoreValve overlap with long-term data from the US CoreValve High Risk Study, which reported major stroke rates of 3.9% at 30 days, 5.8% at 1 year, and 6.8% at 2 years.[9] In the FORWARD study, major stroke rates with the new-generation Evolut R were considerably lower, with 1.8% at 30 days and 2.1% at 1 year.[12,18] The PARTNER-II trial reported major stroke rates with the Sapien XT valve of 3.2% at 30 days, 5.0% at 1 year, and 6.2% at 2 years.[13] In a large propensity-matched analysis in which the Sapien 3 valve was used, major stroke occurred less frequently, with 1.0% at 30 days and 2.3% at 1 year.[14] Also, in the PARTNER-II Sapien 3 registry, lower stroke rates were

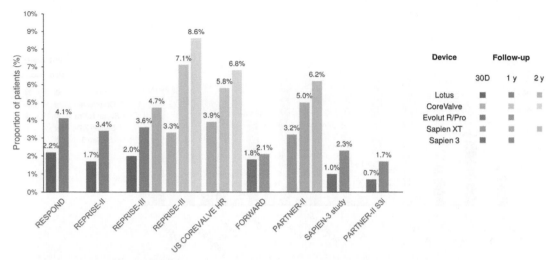

Fig. 5. Major stroke rates at 30 days, 1 year, and 2 years across large trials.

reported compared with its predecessor, namely 0.7% at 30 days and 1.7% at 1 year.

At present, the causal link between embolic debris and the occurrence of neurologic events is undisputed.[19] Recently, a study by Seeger and colleagues[20] showed that less embolic debris was captured by the Sentinel cerebral protection device after implantation of the Lotus valve compared with Evolut R and Sapien 3. Hypothetically, this might be the result of the gradual expansion of the Lotus valve in contrast with the rapid expansion of the self-expanding CoreValve and the even more rapid balloon-expandable Sapien 3 valve. Moreover, the need for postdilatation with these valves might aggravate this effect. Nevertheless, it seems implausible that a future valve would not initiate any embolic debris and therefore it is likely that the solution to eliminate cerebral complications lies not within a valve design but in avoiding the debris entering the brain; for instance, by the use of cerebral protection devices.

Paravalvular Leak

The Lotus valve is eminently suited for eliminating PVL because of its adaptive seal, which conforms to aortic root irregularities, as well as the possibility for full device repositioning or retrieval on complete deployment if the initial implantation is unacceptable. An overview of PVL rates in large TAVR trials is shown in **Fig. 6**. The REPRISE-II study reported the following rates of PVL at 30 days with the Lotus valve: mild in 16.8% and moderate/severe in 1.0%. In REPRISE-III, moderate or severe PVL at 30 days of follow-up was noted in 0.6% and mild in 10.7% within the Lotus group compared

with moderate or severe PVL in 7.2% and mild in 48.7% within the CoreValve group.[6] In the RESPOND postmarket registry, PVL as assessed by echocardiography at hospital discharge was adjudicated by an independent core laboratory. PVL was absent or trace in 92.0%, mild in 7.7%, moderate in 0.3%, and severe PVL did not occur. These surgerylike numbers have not been reproduced with any of the other THV platforms. The US CoreValve High Risk Study reported paravalvular regurgitation at 30 days with the CoreValve as mild in 35.7% and moderate/severe in 9.0%.[9] In the SURTAVI-trial, results of TAVR with the CoreValve were compared with SAVR.[11] At discharge, PVL occurred more frequently with CoreValve than with SAVR, being mild in 33.7% and 4.3% and moderate in 3.4% and 0.3%, respectively. The FORWARD study reported PVL at discharge after TAVR with the Evolut R valve, being mild in 30.9%, and moderate/severe in 1.9%.[18] In the Evolut low-risk trial, patients at low surgical risk were randomized between TAVR with the Evolut R/Pro valve or SAVR.[4] At 30 days, PVL was reported as mild in 36.0% versus 3.0%, and moderate/severe in 3.4% versus 0.4%, respectively. The Source 3 registry reported PVL at 30 days with the Sapien 3 valve, with mild in 23.3% and moderate/severe in 3.1%. The PARTNER-II Sapien 3 registry reported mild PVL in 40.3% and moderate/severe in 3.7%.[21] In the PARTNER-III trial, PVL at 30 days with the Sapien 3 valve was mild in 28.7% and moderate/severe in 0.8%. In the PARTNER-IIA trial, PVL at 30 days with the Sapien XT valve was mild in 22.5% and moderate/severe in 3.7%.[13] Notably, patients with moderate/severe PVL had a higher mortality

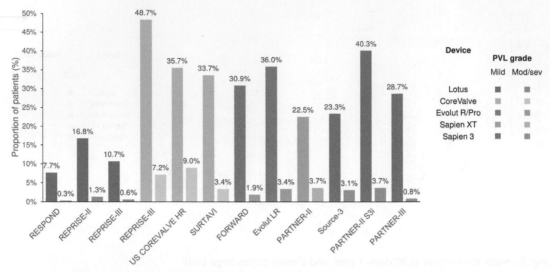

Fig. 6. Paravalvular regurgitation (PVL) at 30 days across larger trials.

compared with those with none/trace, at 2 years of follow-up. The higher mortality was also confirmed by an in-depth analysis from the PARTNER-I trials, which showed higher 1-year mortality and rehospitalization rates associated with moderate/severe PVL (35.1% and 31.3%, respectively), and mild PVL (22.2% and 23.0%, respectively), compared with none/trace (15.9% and 14.4%, respectively).[22]

Hemodynamic Performance

In the REPRISE-II study, early echocardiographic follow-up showed a mean effective orifice area (EOA) of 1.7 cm^2 and a mean gradient of 11.5 mm Hg after Lotus valve implantation.[17] In RESPOND, post-Lotus EOA was 1.8 cm^2 with a mean gradient of 10.8 mm Hg.[16] An in-depth analysis of the hemodynamic performance from the randomized REPRISE-III trial noted a larger EOA 30 days after TAVR with CoreValve compared with Lotus (1.96 cm^2 vs 1.64 cm^2, respectively) and a lower mean gradient (8.19 mm Hg vs 12.26 mm Hg, respectively).[23] In the Lotus group, 8.6% met the criterion for residual valve stenosis compared with 1.2% in the CoreValve group. In both groups, higher gradients did not affect either mortality or functional outcomes (ie, New York Heart Association [NYHA] class and Kansas City Cardiomyopathy Questionnaire score). However, the REPRISE-III study did not report any data on the occurrence of prosthesis-patient mismatch (PPM). It has been shown that high transvalvular gradients might affect clinical outcomes through the PPM phenomenon, in which the EOA is virtually too small for the patient's body size (ie, body surface

area), and thus for the required cardiac output. The cutoff value for PPM is an indexed EOA less than 0.85 cm^2/m^2, moderate PPM between 0.65 and 0.85 cm^2/m^2, and severe PPM less than 0.65 cm^2/m^2. PPM is not rare after TAVR, and seems higher with annular designs (eg, SAPIEN and Lotus) compared with a supra-annular design (eg, Evolut, ACURATE), as has been shown in recent low-risk trials. In the randomized PARTNER-III trial, EOA at 30-day follow-up was similar between TAVR with Sapien 3 and SAVR (1.7 cm^2 vs 1.8 cm^2, respectively), and PPM was common in 62% of patients after TAVR (moderate 54%; severe 8%) and 57% after SAVR (moderate 47%; severe 9%).[3] In the randomized Evolut low-risk trial, EOA at 30-day follow-up was larger in patients treated with TAVR compared with SAVR (2.2 cm^2 vs 2.0 cm^2). Also, PPM after TAVR was noted in only 11% of patients and severe PPM occurred seldom (1%), whereas this was noted in 20% (moderate 16%, severe 4%) of patients treated with SAVR. A recent analysis from the STS/American College of Cardiology (ACC) TVT Registry reported that PPM after TAVR occurred in 37% of patients (moderate in 25%; severe in 12%).[24] Severe PPM was associated with a significantly higher mortality at 1-year follow-up compared with patients without PPM, although the effect was modest (hazard ratio of 1.19 after adjustment for potential confounders). In conclusion, echocardiographic data after TAVR with Lotus suggest a slightly less favorable EOA with this THV, although it is highly questionable whether this results in clinically relevant PPM that could affect clinical or functional outcomes. It seems plausible that the favorable effect on minimizing PVL outweighs the presumed smaller EOA associated with the Lotus THV.

Functional Outcomes

The RESPOND postmarket study showed a marked improvement of functional status in patients treated with Lotus (improvement of 2 or more NYHA functional classes in 35%). Within the randomized REPRISE-III trial, the investigators reported an improvement in NYHA functional class of 2 or more in 37.3% of patients treated with Lotus, compared with 21.3% treated with CoreValve.[7] Ultimately, 30% more patients were asymptomatic after Lotus implantation (ie, NYHA class I) compared with Core-Valve at 2-year follow-up. This enhanced symptomatic relief could be associated with the PVL benefit seen with Lotus, but this hypothesis requires further study.

Conduction Disturbances

The frequent occurrence of newly induced conduction disturbances has become a recognized consequence of TAVR with Lotus and remains its Achilles heel. In the past, conduction disturbances were assigned to the self-expanding designs rather than the balloon-expandable designs,[25] but currently the mechanically expanded Lotus seems to have a significant effect on the conduction system. Large trials consistently reported high incidences of new-onset left bundle branch block and subsequent need for a permanent pacemaker, as shown in **Fig. 7**. In REPRISE-II, the 30-day rate of permanent pacemaker implantation (PPI) was 28.6%.[17] The randomized REPRISE-III trial and the postmarket RESPOND study confirmed this finding (PPI rates of 29.1% and 30.0%, respectively).[6,16] In the control arm of the REPRISE-III trial, the PPI rate associated with CoreValve was 15.8% at 30 days. The US CoreValve High Risk Study reported a PPI rate of 19.8%.[9] With the next-generation self-expanding Evolut R valve, the reported PPI rate was comparable at 17.5%.[18] The transition with the Evolut valve to low-risk patients did not result in lower PPI, as shown by the recently published Evolut low-risk trial, in which 17.4% of patients treated with the Evolut R/Pro underwent PPI versus 6.1% of those treated with SAVR. As mentioned earlier, the PPI rate associated with the balloon-expandable valves tends to be much lower than that observed with self-expanding or mechanically expanding valves. The PARTNER-IIA intermediate-risk study reported a 30-day PPI rate of 8.5% with the Sapien XT valve. Similarly, the PPI rate was 10.2% in the PARTNER-II S3i propensity-matched study, which evaluated the Sapien 3 device in intermediate-risk patients,.[14] In the intermediate-risk subgroup of the Sapien 3 registry, the PPI rate was also similar at 10.1%.[21] The SOURCE 3 registry reported a PPI rate of 12.3% in patients who underwent transfemoral TAVR with the Sapien 3 valve.

Several theories have been proposed to explain the increased incidence of PPI associated with Lotus valve implantation, some of which are related to the implantation technique and some to the device itself. First, there is the process in which the metallic frame foreshortens with subsequent radial expansion in order to perfectly fit the native annulus and create a continuum with the aortic root (as shown in **Fig. 1**).

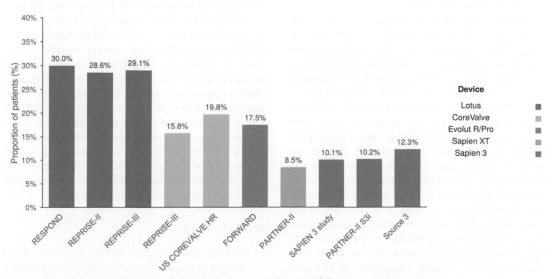

Fig. 7. Permanent pacemaker implantation (PPI) rates at 30-day follow-up across large trials.

Conceivably, this pressure and traction within the aortic root and thus on the membranous septum might induce significant conduction defects. Second, the valve contains a seal that adapts to aortic root irregularities and minimizes PVL, and this might enhance the pressure that is expressed on the conduction bundles. Third, and closely related to the first technical aspect, is that the foreshortening of the valve is difficult to estimate by the operator and thus might result in pragmatically deep implantations with increased contact of the valve frame across the membranous septum and conduction bundles.

The original Lotus valve required deep left ventricular outflow tract (LVOT) interaction because of the foreshortening from both ends that occurred during locking of the valve, as described earlier. A dedicated subanalysis from the RESPOND trial revealed that implantation depth was a major contributor for the need for PPI, with an adjusted odds ratio of 1.20 per millimeter.[26] Hypothetically, a shallower implantation would lead to less LVOT interaction and thus minimize the risk of post-TAVR conduction disturbances and subsequent need for permanent pacing. By only altering the implantation depth, the rate of new permanent pacemakers would come down from more than 40% with deep implants to 20% with shallow implants. The next-generation Lotus valve with Depth Guard technology involves foreshortening of the stent frame from the top down during unsheathing. This foreshortening results in a less deep protrusion of the distal edge of the stent frame into the LVOT. Consequently, LVOT protrusion with Depth Guard is more predictable and less pronounced, resulting in less interaction with the LVOT.

Recently, the RESPOND Extension study reported promising results with the use of the Depth Guard technology.[8] Fifty patients were treated with this new technological iteration of the Lotus valve, which resulted in a PPI rate of 20.0%, compared with 34.6% in the general RESPOND cohort. Although patient numbers are limited, this finding suggests that, with refinement of the valve design and implantation technique, the incidence of PPI might be reduced. Sizing algorithms may also affect the need for PPI. The LVOT tapers down relative to the aortic annulus in up to one-third of patients. The consequence is that a sizing algorithm based solely on annular dimensions would result in enhanced oversizing relative to the LVOT, with concomitantly more pressure trauma on the conduction system. Further reductions in PPI with Lotus may be achieved by revisiting sizing charts and incorporating LVOT dimensions to determine the Lotus size.

Lotus in Complex Anatomy

The repositioning/retrievable capacity and the sealing fabric make Lotus attractive in challenging aortic root anatomies, such as bicuspid aortic valve stenosis and the extremes of aortic root calcification: both heavily calcified valves and valves in which calcium is absent (eg, native aortic valve regurgitation).

With the early-generation valves, TAVR in bicuspid anatomy was plagued by high rates of significant PVL.[27] Although data for Lotus in patients with bicuspid anatomy are scarce, the available data are promising. In a study by Yoon and colleagues,[28] PVL was none or trace in 82%, mild in 18%, and no moderate or severe. With the early-generation CoreValve and Sapien XT, PVL was more common (CoreValve, none/trace 50%, mild 39%, moderate 10%, and severe 2%; Sapien XT, none/trace 57%, mild 37%, and moderate 6%). Results from the RESPOND postmarket registry show that hemodynamic performance of Lotus is comparable between tricuspid and bicuspid aortic valves.[29] There was no and mild PVL in 86% and 14% of cases and moderate or severe PVL was not seen.

SUMMARY

Over the past several years, multiple THV iterations created an interesting range of options with which to perform TAVR. The Lotus valve has several attractive features that make it intuitive and easy to use, even for operators at the beginning of their procedural experience. The ability to eradicate even mild PVL mirrors the outcomes of SAVR. The incidence of stroke seems to be acceptably low and functional outcomes (ie, NYHA functional status) remain excellent over time. Conduction disturbances represent the Lotus valve's Achilles heel and are relevant particularly in young patients at low surgical risk. New design iterations of the Lotus valve and refined sizing algorithms may help mitigate the need for PPI and consolidate its best-in-class results in terms of PVL. Ongoing trials with the Lotus Edge THV are ongoing and should help define the safety and efficacy of the Lotus transcatheter heart valve in contemporary practice.

REFERENCES

1. Baumgartner H, Falk V, Bax JJ, et al. 2017 ESC/EACTS Guidelines for the management of valvular heart disease. Eur Heart J 2017;38:2739–91.

2. Nishimura RA, Otto CM, Bonow RO, et al. 2014 AHA/ACC guideline for the management of patients with valvular heart disease: a report of the American College of Cardiology/American Heart Association task force on practice guidelines. Circulation 2014;129:e521–643.

3. Mack MJ, Leon MB, Thourani VH, et al. Transcatheter aortic-valve replacement with a balloon-expandable valve in low-risk patients. N Engl J Med 2019;380(18):1695–705.

4. Popma JJ, Deeb GM, Yakubov SJ, et al. Transcatheter aortic-valve replacement with a self-expanding valve in low-risk patients. N Engl J Med 2019; 380(18):1706–15.

5. Meredith IT, Walters DL, Dumonteil N, et al. 1-year outcomes with the fully repositionable and retrievable lotus transcatheter aortic replacement valve in 120 high-risk surgical patients with severe aortic stenosis: results of the REPRISE II study. JACC Cardiovasc Interv 2016;9:376–84.

6. Feldman TE, Reardon MJ, Rajagopal V, et al. Effect of mechanically expanded vs self-expanding transcatheter aortic valve replacement on mortality and major adverse clinical events in High-risk patients with aortic stenosis: the REPRISE III randomized clinical trial. JAMA 2018;319:27–37.

7. Reardon MJ, Feldman TE, Meduri CU, et al. Two-year outcomes after transcatheter aortic valve replacement with mechanical vs self-expanding valves: the REPRISE III randomized clinical trial. JAMA Cardiol 2019. https://doi.org/10.1001/jamacardio.2019.0091.

8. Van Mieghem NM, Wohrle J, Hildick-Smith D, et al. Use of a repositionable and fully retrievable aortic valve in routine clinical practice: the RESPOND Study and RESPOND extension cohort. JACC Cardiovasc Interv 2019;12:38–49.

9. Adams DH, Popma JJ, Reardon MJ, et al. Transcatheter aortic-valve replacement with a self-expanding prosthesis. N Engl J Med 2014;370: 1790–8.

10. Reardon MJ, Adams DH, Kleiman NS, et al. 2-year outcomes in patients undergoing surgical or self-expanding transcatheter aortic valve replacement. J Am Coll Cardiol 2015;66:113–21.

11. Reardon MJ, Van Mieghem NM, Popma JJ, et al. Surgical or transcatheter aortic-valve replacement in intermediate-risk patients. N Engl J Med 2017; 376:1321–31.

12. Manoharan G, Van Mieghem NM, Windecker S, et al. 1-year outcomes with the evolut R self-expanding transcatheter aortic valve: from the International FORWARD Study. JACC Cardiovasc Interv 2018;11:2326–34.

13. Leon MB, Smith CR, Mack MJ, et al. Transcatheter or surgical aortic-valve replacement in intermediate-risk patients. N Engl J Med 2016;374:1609–20.

14. Thourani VH, Kodali S, Makkar RR, et al. Transcatheter aortic valve replacement versus surgical valve replacement in intermediate-risk patients: a propensity score analysis. Lancet 2016;387: 2218–25.

15. Wendler O, Schymik G, Treede H, et al. SOURCE 3: 1-year outcomes post-transcatheter aortic valve implantation using the latest generation of the balloon-expandable transcatheter heart valve. Eur Heart J 2017;38:2717–26.

16. Falk V, Wohrle J, Hildick-Smith D, et al. Safety and efficacy of a repositionable and fully retrievable aortic valve used in routine clinical practice: the RESPOND Study. Eur Heart J 2017;38:3359–66.

17. Meredith Am IT, Walters DL, Dumonteil N, et al. Transcatheter aortic valve replacement for severe symptomatic aortic stenosis using a repositionable valve system: 30-day primary endpoint results from the REPRISE II study. J Am Coll Cardiol 2014;64:1339–48.

18. Grube E, Van Mieghem NM, Bleiziffer S, et al. Clinical outcomes with a repositionable self-expanding transcatheter aortic valve prosthesis: the International FORWARD Study. J Am Coll Cardiol 2017;70:845–53.

19. Van Mieghem NM, Schipper ME, Ladich E, et al. Histopathology of embolic debris captured during transcatheter aortic valve replacement. Circulation 2013;127:2194–201.

20. Seeger J, Virmani R, Romero M, et al. Significant differences in debris captured by the sentinel dual-filter cerebral embolic protection during transcatheter aortic valve replacement among different valve types. JACC Cardiovasc Interv 2018;11:1683–93.

21. Kodali S, Thourani VH, White J, et al. Early clinical and echocardiographic outcomes after SAPIEN 3 transcatheter aortic valve replacement in inoperable, high-risk and intermediate-risk patients with aortic stenosis. Eur Heart J 2016;37:2252–62.

22. Kodali S, Pibarot P, Douglas PS, et al. Paravalvular regurgitation after transcatheter aortic valve replacement with the Edwards sapien valve in the PARTNER trial: characterizing patients and impact on outcomes. Eur Heart J 2015;36:449–56.

23. Asch FM, Vannan MA, Singh S, et al. Hemodynamic and echocardiographic comparison of the lotus and corevalve transcatheter aortic valves in patients with high and extreme surgical risk: an analysis from the REPRISE III Randomized Controlled Trial. Circulation 2018;137:2557–67.

24. Herrmann HC, Daneshvar SA, Fonarow GC, et al. Prosthesis-patient mismatch in patients undergoing transcatheter aortic valve replacement: from the STS/ACC TVT registry. J Am Coll Cardiol 2018;72:2701–11.

25. Siontis GC, Juni P, Pilgrim T, et al. Predictors of permanent pacemaker implantation in patients with severe aortic stenosis undergoing TAVR: a meta-analysis. J Am Coll Cardiol 2014;64:129–40.

26. van Gils L, Wohrle J, Hildick-Smith D, et al. Importance of contrast aortography with lotus transcatheter aortic valve replacement: a post hoc analysis from the RESPOND post-market study. JACC Cardiovasc Interv 2018;11:119–28.

27. Mylotte D, Lefevre T, Sondergaard L, et al. Transcatheter aortic valve replacement in bicuspid aortic valve disease. J Am Coll Cardiol 2014;64:2330–9.

28. Yoon SH, Lefevre T, Ahn JM, et al. Transcatheter aortic valve replacement with early- and new-generation devices in bicuspid aortic valve stenosis. J Am Coll Cardiol 2016;68:1195–205.

29. Blackman DJ, Van Gils L, Bleiziffer S, et al. Clinical outcomes of the Lotus Valve in patients with bicuspid aortic valve stenosis: an analysis from the RESPOND study. Catheter Cardiovasc Interv 2019;93(6):1116–23.

Conduction System Abnormalities After Transcatheter Aortic Valve Replacement

Mechanism, Prediction, and Management

Gregory L. Judson, MD, Harsh Agrawal, MD, RPVI, FSCAI,
Vaikom S. Mahadevan, MD, FRCP, FSCAI*

KEYWORDS

- TAVR - Transcatheter aortic valve replacement - Aortic stenosis - Conduction abnormalities
- Pacemaker - Heart block

KEY POINTS

- Conduction abnormalities are common following transcatheter aortic valve replacement (TAVR), as the anatomy of the left ventricular and aortic outflow tracts predispose to damage to the conduction system during and after the procedure.
- Patient factors, procedural characteristics, and the type of valve used during TAVR all contribute to the need for permanent pacemaker.
- Careful monitoring of patients post-TAVR can help identify the patients who will require a pacemaker and minimize potential deleterious effects.
- A decision-making algorithm incorporating preexisting conduction abnormalities and electrophysiology testing may improve the appropriate use of permanent pacemakers post-TAVR.

INTRODUCTION

Aortic stenosis (AS) is a common form of valvular heart disease, the global burden of which continues to increase.[1] Untreated, severe symptomatic AS carries a high mortality rate.[2] Initially performed in patients deemed unsuitable for surgery, and then advancing to become an option for patients with high, intermediate, and now low operative risk, transcatheter aortic valve replacement (TAVR) has revolutionized the treatment of symptomatic severe AS and is deemed noninferior to surgical aortic valve replacement (SAVR) with regard to mortality at 1 year.[3–7] Although TAVR is associated with lower rates of certain periprocedural

complications compared with SAVR, in the landmark TAVR trials, the need for permanent pacemaker (PPM) implantation after TAVR was generally higher compared with SAVR.

Currently, the 2 TAVR devices in clinical use in the United States are the Sapien (Edwards Lifesciences, Irvine, CA, USA) and the Evolut (Medtronic, Santa Rosa, CA, USA) systems. The Sapien 3 valve is a balloon-expandable system with bovine pericardial tissue leaflets, a cobalt-chromium frame, and lower fabric skirt that sits in the intravalvular position. The Evolut is a self-expanding, porcine pericardial tissue valve with a nitinol frame that is anchored in the supravalvular/supra-annular position. The lower

---

Division of Cardiology, University of California, San Francisco, 505 Parnassus Avenue, L524, San Francisco, CA 94143, USA
* Corresponding author.
E-mail address: Vaikom.mahadevan@ucsf.edu

Intervent Cardiol Clin 8 (2019) 403–409
https://doi.org/10.1016/j.iccl.2019.06.003
2211-7458/19/© 2019 Elsevier Inc. All rights reserved.

portion of the Medtronic system sits in the left ventricular outflow tract (LVOT) and exerts a higher radial force.[8] The latest generation of this transcatheter valve, the Evolut Pro, is similar in design and implantation to the Evolut R, but has an outer wrap of porcine pericardium to help minimize perivalvular leak.

In a meta-analysis of patients undergoing TAVR, the most common indications for PPM implantation were complete atrioventricular (AV) block, second-degree type II AV block, sick sinus syndrome, left bundle branch block (LBBB) with first-degree AV block, atrial fibrillation with slow response/complete AV block, alternating right bundle branch block (RBBB)/LBBB, and sinus bradycardia.[9] The rates of post-TAVR conduction abnormalities requiring a PPM range from 4.3% to 43% with self-expanding valves associated with a higher rates of PPM implantation than balloon-expandable valves, and newer valve systems having lower rates than earlier generation valves.[10–12] The recent generation self-expanding CoreValve Evolut R has a PPM rate of 14.7% to 17.4%, whereas the Sapien 3 has a PPM rate of 6.5% to 12.3% with optimal positioning.[6,7,13,14] The newest generation Evolut Pro valve seems to have similar rates of PPM implantation as the Evolut R.[15]

Recent data suggest the safety and efficacy of TAVR in low-risk patient cohorts using self-expanding and balloon-expandable valves. In the PARTNER 3 (placement of aortic transcatheter valve 3) trial of the balloon-expandable Sapien 3 valve, the rate of new LBBB was significantly higher in the TAVR group compared with SAVR (23.7% vs 8%, P<.001), but the rates of new PPM were not significantly different between the 2 treatment arms at 30 days (6.6% vs 4.1%, P = .09) or at 1 year (7.3% vs 5.4%, P = .24).[6] In the Evolut Low Risk trial, the rate of new pacemaker implantation with the self-expanding supra-annular prosthesis system was significantly higher compared with SAVR at 30 days (17.4% vs 6.1%, 95% credible interval for difference: 8.0%–14.7%).[7] These data are in line with previous studies implicating self-expanding valves with higher rates of PPM than their balloon-expandable counterparts.

Although the rates of PPM implantation have decreased with each successive iteration of TAVR valves, an understanding of the mechanisms, risk factors, and management options for patients who experience conduction abnormalities following TAVR is essential for all cardiologists who care for these patients.

MECHANISMS OF CONDUCTION ABNORMALITIES FOLLOWING TRANSCATHETER AORTIC VALVE REPLACEMENT

A detailed explanation of the mechanisms that underlie post-TAVR conduction abnormalities requires a brief overview of the anatomic structures in and around the aortic root and the LVOT, because the conduction system of the heart lies in close proximity to these structures. The aortic root is made up of the sinuses of Valsalva, the fibrous interleaflet triangles, and the valvar leaflets themselves.[16] It is a direct extension of the LVOT, which is itself composed of muscular components (the ventricular septum) and fibrous components (the continuity between the leaflets of the aortic and mitral valves).

The AV node is located within Koch's triangle, an anatomic area within the right atrium bounded by the tendon of Todaro, the attachment of the septal leaflet of the tricuspid valve, and the orifice of the coronary sinus.[8] The AV node continues as the His-bundle through the membranous septum. There is heterogeneity in the location of the AV node, with ~50% of patients exhibiting a predominantly right-sided AV node, ~30% with a left-sided orientation, and the remaining ~20% of patients with an AV node running under the membranous septum just below the endocardium. The latter 2 anatomic variants may predispose patients to increased risk of conduction abnormalities following TAVR.[17]

The left bundle branch emerges from beneath the membranous septum and is located within the interventricular septum, close to the base of the interleaflet triangle that separates the noncoronary and the right coronary leaflets of the aortic valve.[18] This relationship of the left bundle to the aortic root explains why LBBB is the most common conduction system abnormality following TAVR, as the valve itself can exert direct pressure on the conduction system (Fig. 1). If LBBB does occur post-TAVR, it appears before hospital discharge in most cases, and increases the risk of PPM implantation. It does not appear to increase overall mortality in some studies,[19,20] although the data are conflicting, as other studies have suggested an increase in mortality with LBBB post-TAVR.[21,22]

PREDICTION OF CONDUCTION SYSTEM ABNORMALITIES POSTTRANSCATHETER AORTIC VALVE REPLACEMENT

Preprocedural patient characteristics and peri-procedural considerations are important

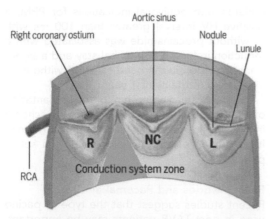

Fig. 1. Spatial relationship between the 3 cusps of the aortic valve and the zone where the left bundle branch emerges beneath the membranous septum. L, left cusp; NC, noncoronary cusp; RCA, right coronary artery. (*From* Mangieri A et al. TAVI and Post Procedural Cardiac Conduction Abnormalities. *Front Cardiovasc Med.* 2018;5; with permission.)

predictors for conduction system abnormalities following TAVR. In a large meta-analysis that included a mix of balloon-expandable and self-expanding systems implanted predominantly via the transfemoral approach, male sex, preprocedural electrocardiographic abnormalities including first-degree AV block, left-anterior hemiblock, and RBBB were significantly associated with the need for PPM. The presence of AV block during the procedure and the use of the self-expanding prosthesis were also associated with an increased need for PPM. The higher rates of conduction system abnormalities observed with the self-expanding transcatheter heart valve compared with the balloon-expandable system may be because of the increased radial force it delivers to the LVOT.[23,24]

In an analysis of 9785 patients undergoing TAVR across 229 sites in the United States between 2011 and 2014 as part of the Society of Thoracic Surgeons (STS)/American College of Cardiology Transcatheter Valve Therapy Registry, patient characteristics associated with higher rates of PPM included increasing age, higher STS Predicted Risk of Operative Mortality score, previous aortic valve procedures, chronic lung disease, and the need for home oxygen. Electrocardiographic, anatomic, and procedural characteristics associated with an increased need for PPM were conduction defects on the preprocedural electrocardiogram, larger aortic annulus size and valve area, need for a larger prosthesis, and the use of valve oversizing.[10] Preoperative atrial fibrillation, left-posterior

hemiblock, LBBB, and ejection fraction were not associated with the need for PPM.

Recent studies have also implicated post-TAVR balloon dilation, a method used to treat insufficiently expanded valves and/or significant perivalvular leak, as a significant predictor of PPM.[25] This same study also found PR prolongation greater than 178 ms post-TAVR as an important risk factor for PPM.

Given the proximity of the conduction system to the LVOT and aortic root, the positioning of the TAVR valve has been shown to influence the rate of rhythm disturbances after implantation. Depth of the prosthesis within the LVOT, as measured by the mean distance from the annular margin of the noncoronary cusp to the ventricular end of the prosthesis on computed tomography, is a significant predictor of PPM implantation: patients requiring a PPM had a mean depth of 9.7 ± 4.1 mm, compared with versus 6.3 ± 3.4 mm among patients who did not require a PPM.[26] A cutoff of 6 mm depth of the TAVR valve into the LVOT was also suggested as a useful predictor of PPM in the ADVANCE II trial using the CoreValve self-expanding prosthesis.[27] Valve depth within the LVOT also seems to be an important predictor of PPM use with the balloon-expandable system. The Sapien 3 valve includes an external tissue seal on the ventricular side of the valve that is meant to minimize perivalvular leak. However, this valve is 3 to 4 mm longer than its predecessor, the Sapien XT, and therefore can extend deeper into the LVOT. In 1 study, the Sapien 3 was noted to have higher rates of PPM than the Sapien XT; however, this rate decreased to a level similar to that of the XT valve with optimal positioning, and the Sapien 3 was associated with very low rates of PPM use in the patients treated at experienced centers within the PARTNER 3 trial.[6,14]

Most conduction system problems following TAVR occur within the first 48 hours after the procedure. However, a minority of patients may develop late conduction disease. RBBB and an increase in the PR interval have been identified as independent predictors of delayed advanced conduction disturbances requiring PPM.[18] Preexisting RBBB has been shown to be a predictor of increased cardiovascular mortality after TAVR as well, and hence such patients need careful follow-up surveillance post-TAVR.[28]

MANAGEMENT AND CLINICAL IMPLICATIONS

The long-term deleterious consequences of ventricular pacing are well known. In TAVR, PPM implantation has been associated with an increased risk for heart failure hospitalization, all-cause readmission, emergency department visits, days spent in the intensive care unit, overall length of stay, maintenance of a persistently reduced ejection fraction, and overall mortality.[29–31] This risk may be particularly increased among patients with already reduced ejection fraction.[32]

One of the limitations of studies that evaluate the incidence of PPM implantation following TAVR is the heterogeneity in clinical indications for PPM placement and uncertainty regarding the timing and definitive indications for PPM. The duration of the PR interval has been shown to peak on post-TAVR days 4 to 6 and the QRS duration on days 7 to 9.[33] In the PARTNER registry, the mean time to PPM implantation was 4.1 days.[19] Even among patients who experience high-degree AV block following TAVR, electrical recovery can eventually occur in 22% to 56% of patients.[34,35] Increased PR interval and preexisting RBBB are reliable predictors of the long-term need for pacing, whereas LBBB and QRS width is not.

In patients without a preexisting bundle branch block or PPM, new RBBB or PPM implantation was associated with increased all-cause mortality greater than 1 year from TAVR implantation.[36] Development of either condition was also associated with an increased risk of heart failure hospitalization and reduced left ventricular ejection fraction. New LBBB with reduced left ventricular ejection fraction has been implicated in an increased risk of sudden death after TAVR.[37] In a substudy of the PARTNER trial, the presence of a new or old PPM or new bundle branch block was associated with higher mortality and increased risk of rehospitalizations.[38] It is hypothesized that lack of left ventricle synchrony owing to right ventricle pacing or LBBB, shortening of diastole, and abnormal septal motion can reduce ejection fraction over time and precipitate heart failure.[39]

Recent data from the PARTNER 2 registry of 3763 patients failed to show any relationship between pacemaker implantation post-TAVR and survival at 1 year, or an improvement in quality-of-life.[40] More data are needed to validate this finding, which differs from other studies.

Additional Testing and Practical Considerations

Electrophysiology studies can also be helpful in determining the need for PPM post-TAVR. Ideally, an electrophysiology study would be able to identify those patients who do not require long-term ventricular pacing.[41] Among

patients with equivocal indications for PPM, a positive HV interval greater than 100 ms with or without procainamide was associated with a reduction in length of hospital stay and a significant reduction in the need for PPM without an increase in mortality at 1 year.[31]

We propose an algorithm for the implantation of PPM following TAVR (Fig. 2). This schema incorporates preexisting conduction abnormalities with an electrophysiology study in select patients.

Pacing Modes and Pacemaker Types

Recent studies suggest that the type of pacing used in post-TAVR patients may be important. In a multicenter study involving 1621 patients who underwent TAVR, of whom 16.4% received a PPM, a retrospective analysis was undertaken to determine the effect of various pacing programming modes on clinical outcomes. During a follow-up period of 13 months, 53% of patients were pacemaker dependent (defined as the absence or inadequate ventricular rhythm >95% of the time on pacemaker interrogation). Conventional dual-chamber pacing (DDD) mode was associated with higher rates of pacemaker dependency compared with other modes aimed at optimizing native conduction (namely AAI/DDD or VVI modes). Heart failure hospitalizations were significantly increased in the DDD group (81.8% vs 54.6%, P = .03), and there was a trend to increased overall mortality in this group (73% vs 96%, P = .06).[42] Along with pacing modes aimed at encouraging native conduction, cardiac resynchronization therapy or His-bundle pacing may be options for reducing the risk of heart failure in patients undergoing TAVR who require a PPM.[43]

Cardiac resynchronization therapy should be considered for patients with a reduced ejection fraction who will have a high pacer burden and a wide LBBB.[43] Leadless pacemakers may be an option for elderly or frail patients in whom dual-chamber pacing is not required and who may not have a high pacemaker burden.[44]

SUMMARY

Conduction disturbances are frequent following TAVR given the location of the cardiac conduction system relative to the site of transcatheter heart valve implantation. Several clinical, anatomic, electrocardiographic, and procedural characteristics are predictors for the need for PPM following TAVR. Care should be taken to limit the use of PPM given the deleterious consequences of pacing post-TAVR, and input from

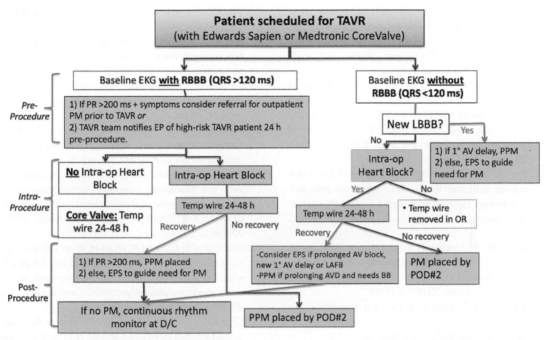

Fig. 2. A proposed decision-making algorithm for permanent pacemaker implantation following transcatheter aortic valve replacement.

electrophysiology specialists should be undertaken to ensure the appropriate use of PPM and optimal pacing methods.

ACKNOWLEDGMENTS

Dr V.S. Mahadevan is a Principal investigator for research studies with Edwards Life Sciences.

REFERENCES

1. Nkomo VT, Gardin JM, Skelton TN, et al. Burden of valvular heart diseases: a population-based study. Lancet 2006;368(9540):1005–11.
2. Turina J, Hess O, Sepulcri F, et al. Spontaneous course of aortic valve disease. Eur Heart J 1987; 8(5):471–83.
3. Leon MB, Smith CR, Mack M, et al. Transcatheter aortic-valve implantation for aortic stenosis in patients who cannot undergo surgery. N Engl J Med 2010;363(17):1597–607.
4. Smith CR, Leon MB, Mack MJ, et al. Transcatheter versus surgical aortic-valve replacement in high-risk patients. N Engl J Med 2011;364(23):2187–98.
5. Leon MB, Smith CR, Mack MJ, et al. Transcatheter or surgical aortic-valve replacement in intermediate-risk patients. N Engl J Med 2016; 374(17):1609–20.
6. Mack MJ, Leon MB, Thourani VH, et al. Transcatheter aortic-valve replacement with a balloon-expandable valve in low-risk patients.

N Engl J Med 2019. https://doi.org/10.1056/ NEJMoa1814052.
7. Popma JJ, Deeb GM, Yakubov SJ, et al. Transcatheter aortic-valve replacement with a self-expanding valve in low-risk patients. N Engl J Med 2019. https://doi.org/10.1056/NEJMoa1816885.
8. Lee JJ, Goldschlager N, Mahadevan VS. Atrioventricular and intraventricular block after transcatheter aortic valve implantation. J Interv Card Electrophysiol 2018;52(3):315–22.
9. Siontis GCM, Jüni P, Pilgrim T, et al. Predictors of permanent pacemaker implantation in patients with severe aortic stenosis undergoing TAVR: a meta-analysis. J Am Coll Cardiol 2014;64(2):129–40.
10. Fadahunsi OO, Olowoyeye A, Ukaigwe A, et al. Incidence, predictors, and outcomes of permanent pacemaker implantation following transcatheter aortic valve replacement: analysis from the U.S. Society of Thoracic Surgeons/American College of Cardiology TVT Registry. JACC Cardiovasc Interv 2016;9(21):2189–99.
11. Buellesfeld L, Stortecky S, Heg D, et al. Impact of permanent pacemaker implantation on clinical outcome among patients undergoing transcatheter aortic valve implantation. J Am Coll Cardiol 2012; 60(6):493–501.
12. AV Block and PPM Implantation in TAVR. American College of Cardiology. Available at: https://www. acc.org/latest-in-cardiology/articles/2017/06/13/07/ 13/av-block-and-ppm-implantation-in-tavr. Accessed February 21, 2019.

13. Kalra SS, Firoozi S, Yeh J, et al. Initial experience of a second-generation self-expanding transcatheter aortic valve: the UK & Ireland Evolut R Implanters' Registry. JACC Cardiovasc Interv 2017;10(3): 276–82.

14. De Torres-Alba F, Kaleschke G, Diller GP, et al. Changes in the pacemaker rate after transition from Edwards SAPIEN XT to SAPIEN 3 transcatheter aortic valve implantation: the critical role of valve implantation height. JACC Cardiovasc Interv 2016;9(8):805–13.

15. Forrest JK, Mangi AA, Popma JJ, et al. Early outcomes with the Evolut PRO repositionable self-expanding transcatheter aortic valve with pericardial wrap. JACC Cardiovasc Interv 2018;11(2): 160–8.

16. Piazza N, de Jaegere P, Schultz C, et al. Anatomy of the aortic valvar complex and its implications for transcatheter implantation of the aortic valve. Circ Cardiovasc Interv 2008;1(1):74–81.

17. Kawashima T, Sato F. Visualizing anatomical evidences on atrioventricular conduction system for TAVI. Int J Cardiol 2014;174(1):1–6.

18. Mangieri A, Montalto C, Pagnesi M, et al. TAVI and post procedural cardiac conduction abnormalities. Front Cardiovasc Med 2018;5. https://doi.org/10.3389/fcvm.2018.00085.

19. Nazif TM, Williams MR, Hahn RT, et al. Clinical implications of new-onset left bundle branch block after transcatheter aortic valve replacement: analysis of the PARTNER experience. Eur Heart J 2014; 35(24):1599–607.

20. Testa L, Latib A, De Marco F, et al. Clinical impact of persistent left bundle-branch block after transcatheter aortic valve implantation with CoreValve Revalving System. Circulation 2013; 127(12):1300–7.

21. Houthuizen P, Van Garsse LAFM, Poels TT, et al. Left bundle-branch block induced by transcatheter aortic valve implantation increases risk of death. Circulation 2012;126(6):720–8.

22. Schymik G, Tzamalis P, Bramlage P, et al. Clinical impact of a new left bundle branch block following TAVI implantation: 1-year results of the TAVIK cohort. Clin Res Cardiol 2015;104(4):351–62.

23. Abdel-Wahab M, Mehilli J, Frerker C, et al. Comparison of balloon-expandable vs self-expandable valves in patients undergoing transcatheter aortic valve replacement: the CHOICE randomized clinical trial. JAMA 2014;311(15):1503–14.

24. Tzamtzis S, Viquerat J, Yap J, et al. Numerical analysis of the radial force produced by the Medtronic-CoreValve and Edwards-SAPIEN after transcatheter aortic valve implantation (TAVI). Med Eng Phys 2013;35(1):125–30.

25. Tichelbäcker T, Bergau L, Puls M, et al. Insights into permanent pacemaker implantation following TAVR in a real-world cohort. PLoS One 2018; 13(10):e0204503.

26. Kammler J, Blessberger H, Fellner F, et al. Implantation depth measured by 64-slice computed tomography is associated with permanent pacemaker requirement following transcatheter aortic valve implantation with the Core Valve(®) system. J Cardiol 2016;67(6):513–8.

27. Petronio AS, Sinning J-M, Van Mieghem N, et al. Optimal implantation depth and adherence to guidelines on permanent pacing to improve the results of transcatheter aortic valve replacement with the medtronic corevalve system: the corevalve prospective, International, Post-Market ADVANCE-II Study. JACC Cardiovasc Interv 2015;8(6):837–46.

28. Watanabe Y, Kozuma K, Hioki H, et al. Pre-existing right bundle branch block increases risk for death after transcatheter aortic valve replacement with a balloon-expandable valve. JACC Cardiovasc Interv 2016;9(21):2210–6.

29. Chamandi C, Barbanti M, Munoz-Garcia A, et al. Long-term outcomes in patients with new permanent pacemaker implantation following transcatheter aortic valve replacement. JACC Cardiovasc Interv 2018;11(3):301–10.

30. Aljabbary T, Qiu F, Masih S, et al. Association of clinical and economic outcomes with permanent pacemaker implantation after transcatheter aortic valve replacement. JAMA Netw Open 2018; 1(1). https://doi.org/10.1001/jamanetworkopen. 2018.0088.

31. Rogers T, Devraj M, Thomaides A, et al. Utility of invasive electrophysiology studies in patients with severe aortic stenosis undergoing transcatheter aortic valve implantation. Am J Cardiol 2018; 121(11):1351–7.

32. Maeno Y, Abramowitz Y, Israr S, et al. Prognostic impact of permanent pacemaker implantation in patients with low left ventricular ejection fraction following transcatheter aortic valve replacement. J Invasive Cardiol 2019;31(2):E15–22.

33. Bjerre Thygesen J, Loh PH, Cholteesupachai J, et al. Reevaluation of the indications for permanent pacemaker implantation after transcatheter aortic valve implantation. J Invasive Cardiol 2014;26(2): 94–9.

34. van der Boon RMA, Van Mieghem NM, Theuns DA, et al. Pacemaker dependency after transcatheter aortic valve implantation with the self-expanding Medtronic CoreValve System. Int J Cardiol 2013; 168(2):1269–73.

35. Boerlage-Van Dijk K, Kooiman KM, Yong ZY, et al. Predictors and permanency of cardiac conduction disorders and necessity of pacing after transcatheter aortic valve implantation. Pacing Clin Electrophysiol 2014;37(11):1520–9.

36. Jørgensen TH, De Backer O, Gerds TA, et al. Mortality and heart failure hospitalization in patients with conduction abnormalities after transcatheter aortic valve replacement. JACC Cardiovasc Interv 2019;12(1):52–61.

37. Urena M, Webb JG, Eltchaninoff H, et al. Late cardiac death in patients undergoing transcatheter aortic valve replacement: incidence and predictors of advanced heart failure and sudden cardiac death. J Am Coll Cardiol 2015;65(5): 437–48.

38. Dizon JM, Nazif TM, Hess PL, et al. Chronic pacing and adverse outcomes after transcatheter aortic valve implantation. Heart 2015;101(20):1665–71.

39. Zannad F, Huvelle E, Dickstein K, et al. Left bundle branch block as a risk factor for progression to heart failure. Eur J Heart Fail 2007;9(1): 7–14.

40. Arnold SV, Zhang Y, Baron SJ, et al. Impact of short-term complications on mortality and quality of life after transcatheter aortic valve replacement. JACC Cardiovasc Interv 2019;12(4):362–9.

41. Naveh S, Perlman GY, Elitsur Y, et al. Electrocardiographic predictors of long-term cardiac pacing dependency following transcatheter aortic valve implantation. J Cardiovasc Electrophysiol 2017; 28(2):216–23.

42. Takahashi M, Badenco N, Monteau J, et al. Impact of pacemaker mode in patients with atrioventricular conduction disturbance after trans-catheter aortic valve implantation. Catheter Cardiovasc Interv 2018;92(7):1380–6.

43. Meguro K, Lellouche N, Teiger E. Cardiac resynchronization therapy improved heart failure after left bundle branch block during transcatheter aortic valve implantation. J Invasive Cardiol 2012;24(3):132–3.

44. Shikama T, Miura M, Shirai S, et al. Leadless pacemaker implantation following transcatheter aortic valve implantation using SAPIEN 3. Korean Circ J 2018;48(6):534–5.

Intracoronary Lithotripsy for the Treatment of Calcified Plaque

Julian Yeoh, B.Pharm, MBBS, FRACP,
Jonathan Hill, MA, MBChB, FRCP*

KEYWORDS

- Percutaneous coronary intervention • Calcified plaque • Intravascular lithotripsy
- Optical coherence tomography • Stent underexpansion • Rotational atherectomy

---

KEY POINTS

- Intravascular lithotripsy (IVL) has been shown to be a safe and feasible alternative method for coronary calcium modification.
- Indications for the use of IVL include coronary calcification noted on angiographic fluoroscopy, the presence of an undilatable lesion, stent underexpansion, and a heavy calcium burden noted on intravascular imaging.
- There are several advantages of IVL compared with other methods of calcium modification, such as providing a more predictable and controlled means of lesion preparation.
- There are several specific clinical scenarios in which IVL can be advantageous, particularly left main stem intervention and when other methods, such as atherectomy, have not been successful.
- Further clinical research is needed to define the exact benefits of IVL, particularly compared with other currently available modalities to modify calcium, and to determine its cost-effectiveness as an adjunct to percutaneous coronary intervention.

INTRODUCTION

Percutaneous coronary intervention (PCI) with drug-eluting stents has become the dominant mode of coronary revascularization in patients presenting with both stable angina and acute coronary syndromes. However, the presence of coronary arterial calcification increases procedural complexity in PCI and is associated with a high risk of major adverse cardiac events (MACEs).[1] In the contemporary PCI era, in which patients with advanced age and multiple comorbidities are indicated for revascularization, significant coronary calcification is becoming more prevalent and creates a major challenge during intervention.[2] Until recently, methods for coronary calcium modification have included, and were limited to, high-pressure noncompliant balloons, cutting balloons, and atherectomy. The Disrupt-CAD I study has recently shown the benefits of intravascular lithotripsy (IVL) in selected cases.[3] This article discusses the introduction of IVL into PCI techniques, indications for use, and specific examples, including the current evidence available in the literature. It discusses where further research and experience is needed within this area.

Disclosures: Permission was sought from Shockwave Medical for reproduction of **Fig. 1A**. Otherwise all images produced are of original production or are referenced appropriately. The authors have no conflicts of interest to disclose.
King's College Hospital NHS Foundation Trust, London SE59RS, UK
* Corresponding author.
E-mail address: jmhill@nhs.net

Intervent Cardiol Clin 8 (2019) 411–424
https://doi.org/10.1016/j.iccl.2019.06.004

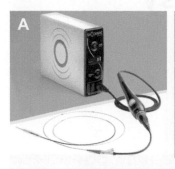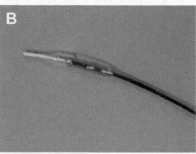

Fig. 1. IVL equipment. (A) Pulse-generating console attached to the wand device used to connect console to lithotripsy balloon. (B) Lithotripsy balloon highlighting the balloon high-energy pulse-generating transducers. (*Courtesy of* Shockwave Medical®, Fremont, CA; with permission.)

PRINCIPLES OF INTRAVASCULAR LITHOTRIPSY IN CORONARY INTERVENTION

Ultrasound energy has been used for more than 30 years in the management of nephrolithiasis in the form of extracorporeal shock wave lithotripsy. More recently, lithotripsy has been incorporated into an intracoronary semicompliant balloon (Shockwave Medical, Fremont, CA). Lithotripsy technology in the coronary arteries for the treatment of coronary calcification was first performed in 2016.[3]

The IVL catheter contains multiple lithotripsy emitters enclosed within a balloon. The emitters convert electrical energy, delivered by an external pulse generator, into transient acoustic circumferential pressure pulses, or sonic pressure waves, that selectively fracture calcium within the vascular plaque, thereby altering vessel compliance.[3] The balloon catheter is advanced to the target lesion in the typical fashion over a standard 0.36-mm (0.014″) coronary guidewire. The balloon is attached to the external pulse generator. After the balloon is inflated at low pressure (4 atm) to avoid barotrauma, a burst of 10 pulses of high energy is delivered over 10 seconds followed by further balloon dilatation (at 6 atm) before deflation of the balloon. This process can be repeated at a target lesion to a total of 8 cycles per balloon (80 pulses). The balloon sizing is based on the desired stent size for that target lesion (ie, 1:1 for the reference vessel diameter) and is often guided by the use of intravascular imaging, which is recommended to guide optimal lesion preparation. Following application of IVL, it is usually recommended that noncompliant balloon dilatation be performed before stent implantation to ensure adequate lesion preparation and ability to dilate the target lesion. The IVL coronary balloons are all 12 mm in length and range from 2.5 mm to 4.0 mm diameter in 0.5-mm increments. All the currently available IVL balloons (Shockwave Medical, Fremont,

CA) have a tip profile of 0.58 mm (0.023″) and a crossing profile of 1.07 mm (0.042″). **Fig. 1** shows the pulse-generating console attached to the wand device used to connect the console to the lithotripsy balloon and the lithotripsy balloon with its high-energy pulse transducers.

INDICATIONS FOR INTRAVASCULAR LITHOTRIPSY

Typical indications for the use of IVL are similar to those for which other methods of coronary calcification should be considered. These indications are summarized in **Box 1** and shown in **Fig. 2**.

CURRENTLY AVAILABLE EVIDENCE FOR INTRAVASCULAR LITHOTRIPSY

The Disrupt-CAD I study was a first-description study presented at the Transcatheter Cardiovascular Therapeutics conference in 2016 and is the pivotal trial for the introduction of IVL into coronary intervention.[3,4] Disrupt-CAD I was a multicenter, prospective, single-arm study of percutaneous lithotripsy before stent implantation in heavily calcified coronary lesions. Patients enrolled included those

---

Box 1
Typical indications for the use of intravascular lithotripsy

- Coronary calcification noted on fluoroscopy or noninvasive imaging (ie, computed tomography coronary angiogram)

- Evidence of an undilatable lesion despite high-pressure noncompliant balloon dilatation as lesion preparation

- Evidence of stent underexpansion, either angiographically or on intravascular imaging

- Evidence of heavy calcification noted on intravascular imaging, either optical coherence tomography or intravascular ultrasonography

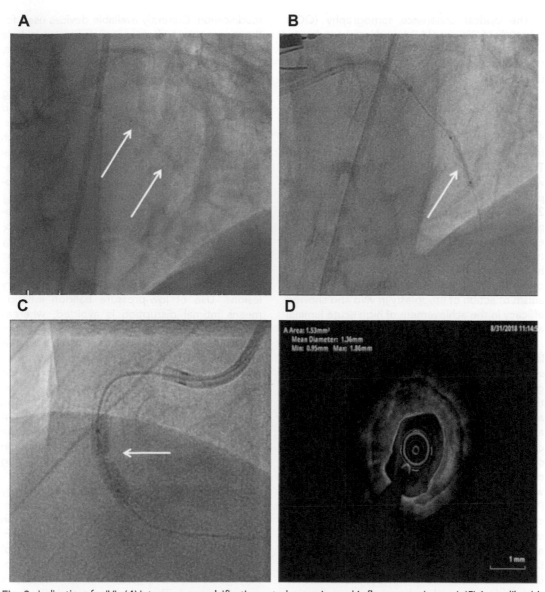

Fig. 2. Indications for IVL. (*A*) Intracoronary calcification noted on angiographic fluoroscopy (*arrows*). (*B*) An undilatable lesion noted despite lesion preparation with a high-pressure noncompliant balloon (*arrow*). (*C*) Stent underexpansion despite postdilatation with a very-high-pressure noncompliant balloon (*arrow*). (*D*) Evidence of circumferential deep calcification noted on optical coherence tomography. (*Courtesy of* Shockwave Medical®, Fremont, CA.)

with stable angina associated with a moderate to severely calcified, de novo coronary lesion of greater than 50% stenosis with a reference vessel diameter between 2.5 and 4.0 mm and of length less than 32 mm. The objective of the study was to assess the safety and performance of the lithoplasty system (Shockwave Medical, Fremont, CA). The primary safety end point was 30-day MACEs and the primary performance end point was clinical success, defined as residual stenosis (<50%) after stenting in the absence of in-hospital MACEs. A total of 60 patients were enrolled. Lithoplasty balloon-based therapy resulted in 98% device success and facilitated 100% stent delivery.[3] The rate of MACEs was 5%, driven by non–Q wave myocardial infarction.[3] Therefore, Disrupt-CAD I showed that lithoplasty seems to be a safe and feasible method of lesion preparation before stenting of complex, calcified, obstructive de novo lesions in patients with stable angina.[3]

The Disrupt-CAD II trial has recently completed recruitment and is currently in its follow-up phase. This postmarket registry seeks to examine the ongoing safety and performance of coronary IVL in heavily calcified coronary lesions in a larger cohort of patents.

The optical coherence tomography (OCT) substudy of Disrupt-CAD I used intravascular imaging to explore the mechanistic effects of the lithoplasty system. The OCT findings of 31 patients were analyzed from the Disrupt-CAD I cohort in whom lithoplasty was used to treat high-grade, severely calcified coronary lesions.[5] Intraplaque calcium fracture was identified in 43% of the lesions, with circumferential, multiple fractures noted in greater than 25% of cases. The frequency of calcium fracture increased with the most severely calcified lesions. The postlithoplasty mean acute area gain was 2.1 mm[2]. After lithoplasty, followed by stent implantation and optimization, the mean stent expansion was 112.0% ± 37.2%.[5] Therefore, this substudy of Disrupt-CAD I showed that high-resolution imaging by OCT delineated calcium modification with fracture as a major mechanism of action of lithoplasty in vivo and showed efficacy in the achievement of high acute luminal area gain to maximize stent expansion.[5]

To date, the evidence for IVL and the published experience have included patients with stable angina with de novo calcified lesions. Our group has presented on extending the application of IVL to a high-risk, real-world population as a safe and feasible alternative to currently available techniques with increasing clinical applicability.[6] This study, which included 54 patients, compared the clinical characteristics and outcomes of those enrolled in the Disrupt-CAD I trial with a clinical cohort of patients undergoing IVL (14 Disrupt-CAD I and 40 clinical). The clinical cohort included patients with acute coronary syndrome (48%), renal replacement therapy (13%), and left main stem and multivessel intervention (28%); 11% of the total cases had a previously undilatable lesion.[6] In this study, there were no cases of device-related coronary perforation and no reflow or 30-day target lesion failure in either group.[6] The OCT substudy of our cohort showed no significant difference in minimal luminal area and mean residual area stenosis in both the Disrupt-CAD I and clinical group, showing that there is increasing clinical applicability of IVL to an all-comers population.[6] Other real-world experience is increasing and has concluded that the IVL device obviates more complex lesion preparation strategies in a broader patient population.[7]

ADVANTAGES AND DISADVANTAGES OF INTRAVASCULAR LITHOTRIPSY

The technology of IVL has several advantages compared with other methods of calcium modification. Currently available devices used for the management of coronary calcification include traditional high-pressure noncompliant balloons, speciality balloons such as cutting and scoring balloons, and atherectomy. High-pressure noncompliant balloons are often ineffective, cutting balloons have a risk of coronary perforation, and there is limited evidence for scoring balloons, which have typically been reserved for side branch bifurcation management.[8] Furthermore, rotational atherectomy has a reported procedural complication rate (a composite of in-hospital death, tamponade, and emergent surgery) of 1.3%.[9]

IVL has been shown to allow calcium modification without affecting the endovascular soft tissue and hence reduces the risk of coronary vessel injury/perforation.[3] The terms soft on soft and hard on hard have been used to describe the use of IVL on calcified intracoronary lesions. Use of low-pressure balloon inflation means intimal disruption is avoided, whereas application of high-energy pulses modifies both superficial and deep calcium.[3] Given this more controlled and predictable means for calcium modification, it reduces the risk of no reflow that is often seen in atherectomy. Given the method of placement of the IVL balloon over a standard guidewire, it allows placement of an additional coronary guidewire down the vessel, which can be useful for lesion preparation of bifurcation lesions, particularly when involving the left main coronary artery.

The major disadvantage of the IVL technology is that the intraballoon pulse-generating technology has made the semicompliant balloon bulky and difficult to deliver to the target lesion, which is already troublesome in the setting of heavy calcification. Therefore, supportive coronary guidewires and guide extension catheters are often used. The advantages and disadvantages of IVL are summarized in Box 2.

SPECIFIC CLINICAL SCENARIOS IN WHICH INTRAVASCULAR LITHOTRIPSY MAY HAVE A DEFINED ROLE

Since IVL has been used for calcium modification in intracoronary lesions there has been an increase in the utility of the technology for specific clinical scenarios. Initial evidence suggested its feasibility and safety in a select group of patients with stable angina and calcified lesions as described in the Disrupt-CAD I study.[3] This study excluded patients with comorbidities that typically increase the risk for calcification, such as previous coronary artery bypass surgery and dependency on renal replacement therapy. The

Box 2
Advantages and disadvantages of intravascular lithotripsy compared with other methods of calcium modification

Advantages

- Provides a more controlled means of calcium modification
- Avoids no reflow as seen in atherectomy
- Allows maintenance of simultaneous guidewire placement for bifurcation lesions (eg, left main stem)
- Has the ability to modify calcification without further vessel injury with minimal trauma on soft tissue
- Less technically demanding compared with atherectomy and hence has a short learning curve to become familiar with the technology

Disadvantages

- Bulky balloon making delivery to the target lesion troublesome (often requiring heavy guidewire and guide extension catheter use)
- May not be able to cross a lesion without the need for atherectomy

authors have presented the utility of the technology in a broader, all-comers group.[6] We concluded that IVL provides a safe and feasible alternative to currently available techniques and shows increasing clinical applicability. Box 3 provides a list of specific scenarios in which IVL has a potential role. An example of each scenario is given later.

Box 3
Specific clinical scenarios in which intravascular lithotripsy has a defined role

1. Undilatable lesions, despite high-pressure balloon dilatation
2. Calcification on intravascular imaging
3. Bifurcation lesion, especially left main coronary artery
4. Stent underexpansion, despite high-pressure balloon dilatation
5. Rotational atherectomy failure
6. Rotational atherectomy facilitated
7. Chronic total occlusion PCI
8. Peripheral use to aid large-bore vascular access; for example, transcatheter aortic valve replacement

Undilatable Lesions

Calcified and undilatable lesions carry risks of stent underexpansion and subsequent restenosis or thrombosis.[10] Traditionally, atherectomy has been the treatment of choice for lesion preparation, particularly where noncompliant balloons, cutting balloons, or so-called buddy cutting balloon techniques have been unsuccessful. IVL has been shown to have a role in this scenario,[11] as shown in **Fig. 3**, in which IVL was used in a lesion in which high-pressure noncompliant balloon pretreatment was unsuccessful. The use of IVL allowed lesion preparation and subsequent stent implantation, with good stent expansion shown on intravascular imaging.

Large Burden of Calcification Shown on Intravascular Imaging

An OCT-based calcium scoring system has recently been developed to identify intracoronary lesions for which lesion preparation with a calcium-modifying adjunct may be beneficial before stent implantation to avoid stent underexpansion.[12] This scoring system incorporates the following OCT-derived target lesion criteria: coronary calcification greater than 180° in circumference, maximal calcium thickness greater than 0.5 mm, and calcium length greater than 5 mm.[12] The use of intravascular imaging to identify these risk factors when fluoroscopic calcification is noted may guide the use of calcium modification, including through IVL. This situation is shown in the case presented in **Fig. 4**, in which OCT was used to identify a lesion with heavy calcification and IVL was used to prepare this lesion before stent implantation. OCT was used before and after IVL, showing calcium fracture as the mechanism of calcium modification.

Bifurcation Lesions, Particularly Left Main Stem

Left main PCI is now a mainstream intervention, with recent data showing similar medium-term outcomes compared with coronary artery bypass grafting.[13,14] Although differences in the longer-term rate of repeat revascularization and nonfatal acute coronary syndrome remain, many patients at high surgical risk are now referred for left main PCI. The immediate mechanical result of left main PCI has a strong influence on outcomes, with the minimum luminal area after PCI correlating strongly with adverse events.[15] This finding has led to the adaptation of the so-called 5, 6, 7, 8 rule as target areas to be achieved in the ostial left circumflex, the left anterior descending, the polygon of confluence, and the left main proximal to the polygon of confluence (**Fig. 5**).

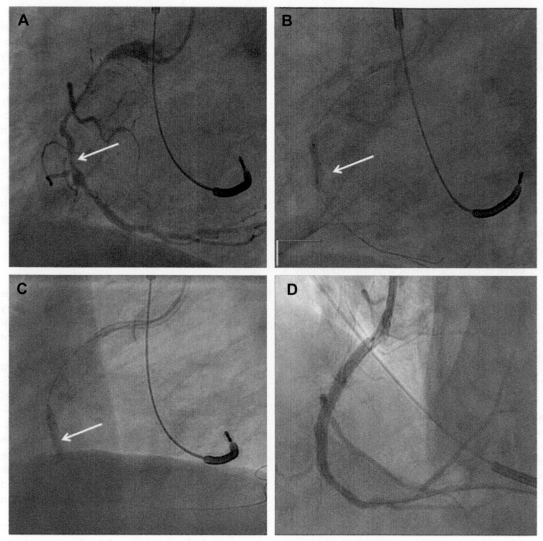

Fig. 3. IVL used in an undilatable lesion. (*A*). Severe mid–right coronary artery (RCA) stenosis (*arrow*). (*B*) Evidence of dog-bone effect (*arrow*) despite high-pressure balloon dilatation. (*C*) Application of IVL with complete balloon expansion (*arrow*). (*D*) Final angiographic result after stent implantation. (*Courtesy of* [C] Shockwave Medical®, Fremont, CA.)

In the presence of a calcified left main lesion, IVL modifies coronary calcification, unlike non-compliant balloon dilatation, restoring vessel compliance, increasing stent expansion, and achieving better stent artery apposition. Compared with atherectomy, IVL allows the maintenance of additional coronary guidewires to allow simultaneous access to the separate daughter vessels, avoiding the risk of acute vessel closure leading to periprocedural myocardial infarction. This technique is particularly useful in the presence of impaired left ventricular function, which often exists in patients with significant left main disease. **Fig. 6** shows a case in which IVL has a defined role in left main disease, making the procedure potentially more effective and safer compared with other methods of calcium modification.

Stent Underexpansion

Stent underexpansion leads to a high incidence of both early adverse outcomes with stent thrombosis and an increased risk of in-stent restenosis leading to subsequent repeat target vessel revascularization.[16,17] Poor lesion preparation is a common mechanism leading to stent underexpansion. Optimal stent expansion can be especially challenging in calcific lesions despite the use of appropriately sized high-pressure noncompliant balloons.[18–20] Furthermore, typical conventional treatment options are limited to high-pressure noncompliant

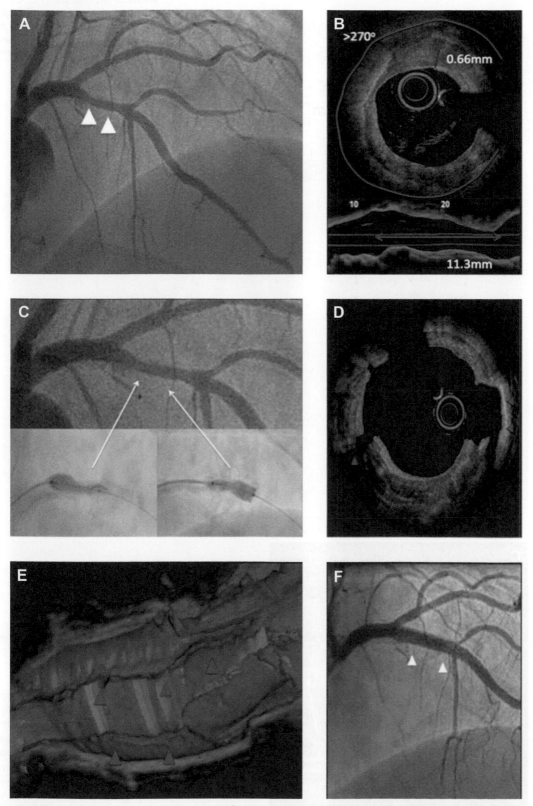

Fig. 4. OCT-guided use of IVL for calcium modification for lesion preparation. (*A*) Severe proximal left anterior descending (LAD) stenosis (*arrowheads*). (*B*) Evidence of circumferential, deep, and long calcification on OCT. (*C*) Application of IVL (*arrows*). (*D*) Evidence of calcium fractures on OCT (*arrowheads*). (*E*) Evidence of calcium fractures/fissures on OCT (*arrowheads*). (*F*) Excellent final angiographic result (*arrowheads*). (*Courtesy of* [*C*] Shockwave Medical®, Fremont, CA.)

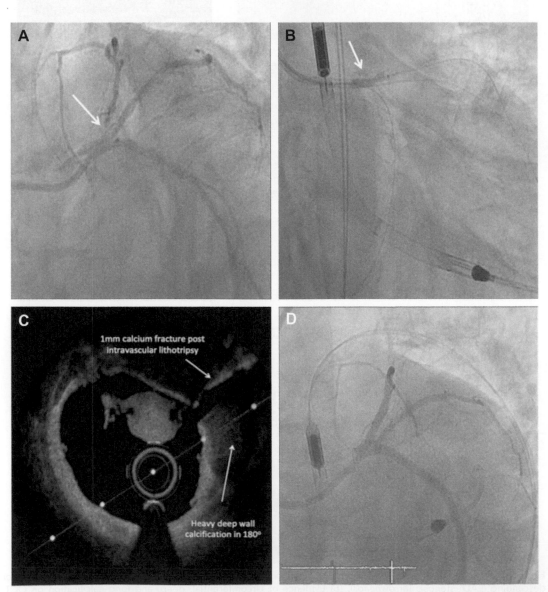

Fig. 5. Minimal stent area cutoff values for left main stem PCI. Cutoff values for the prediction of angiographic in-stent restenosis (ISR) on a segmental basis. LCx, left circumflex artery; LM, left main stem; PoC, polygon of confluence.

LM proximal to PoC 8 mm²

LAD ostium 6 mm²

PoC 7 mm²

LCx ostium 5 mm²

A

B

C

1mm calcium fracture post intravascular lithotripsy

Heavy deep wall calcification in 180°

D

Fig. 6. Left main stem intervention using IVL. (*A*) Severe calcified disease in a trifurcating left main stem including the ostium of the LAD, LCx, and intermediate (*arrow*). (*B*) Application of IVL in the left main stem–LAD junction with maintenance of simultaneous guidewire protecting daughter branches (*arrow*). (*C*) Evidence of calcium fracture in ostial LAD on OCT (*arrows*). (*D*) Excellent final angiographic result; note presence of left ventricular support use during the procedure. (*Courtesy of* [*B*] Shockwave Medical®, Fremont, CA.)

balloon inflation once stent implantation has been performed and there is stent underexpansion despite appropriate inflation pressures.

In the setting of stent underexpansion or where stent underexpansion has led to restenosis, IVL application has become a useful technique to alter vessel compliance by fracturing both the intimal and medial calcification that previously inhibited stent expansion. When IVL is used acutely after stent deployment, the effects on drug delivery and drug polymer characteristics are currently unknown, but may be deleterious. These effects may include issues related to drug polymer integrity and stent integrity leading to future stent corrosion.

Future evaluation of the effects of IVL on drug coating and stent integrity is needed. **Fig. 7** provides an example of IVL being used in an underexpanded stent deployed for the management of in-stent restenosis. Several other cases have recently been published showing the utility of IVL for stent underexpansion.[21,22]

Rotational Atherectomy Failure

Rotational atherectomy for the endovascular treatment of obstructive coronary artery disease emerged in the 1990s and has gained popularity. However, data have not shown long-term benefits on rates of restenosis and MACE, and, being technically more involved, rates even in

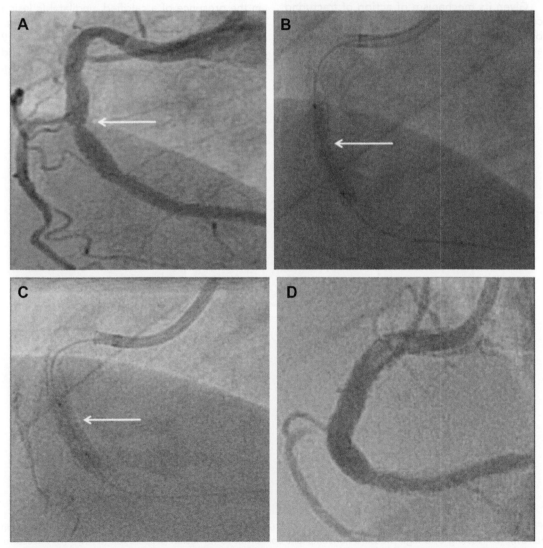

Fig. 7. IVL for stent underexpansion. (*A*) Stent underexpansion after PCI in RCA ISR (*arrow*). (*B*) Wasting of the very-high-pressure balloon (*arrow*). (*C*) Application of IVL in underexpanded segment shows complete balloon dilatation (*arrow*). (*D*) Excellent final angiographic result with complete stent expansion. ([*A, B, C*] *Courtesy of* Shockwave Medical®, Fremont, CA.)

high-volume centers are less than 1%.[23] Rotational atherectomy produces luminal enlargement by physical removal of plaque, reducing plaque rigidity and facilitating vessel dilatation.[23] Rotational atherectomy acts preferentially by ablating hard, inelastic material, such as calcified plaque, that is less able to stretch away from the advancing burr in a process termed differential cutting, which is often determined by wire bias. For this reason, rotational atherectomy may be unsuccessful in debulking the entire burden of calcification in the presence of deep circumferential calcification, and hence may not be able to assist in increasing vessel compliance sufficiently for adequate stent expansion.

Given its mechanism of action of fracturing calcium in a circumferential fashion, IVL may be a suitable alternative where rotational atherectomy has failed to treat the lesion successfully to allow improved lesion compliance.

An example of IVL-facilitated PCI after unsuccessful rotation atherectomy is shown in Fig. 8.

Rotational Atherectomy Facilitated

Placement of the IVL device at the target lesion can be difficult given the bulky nature of the balloon that houses the transducers that generate the ultrasonic energy. Often a heavy guidewire is needed to provide support for delivery to the target lesion. Furthermore, a supportive guide catheter and guide extension catheter may be useful to deliver the balloon to the target lesion. A strategy of rotational atherectomy–facilitated delivery of the IVL balloon to the target lesion has been described in the presence of a calcified, undilatable lesion to which IVL cannot be delivered despite initial predilatation with low-profile balloons. Fig. 9 shows a case in which the initial strategy had been to use the IVL technology to prepare a

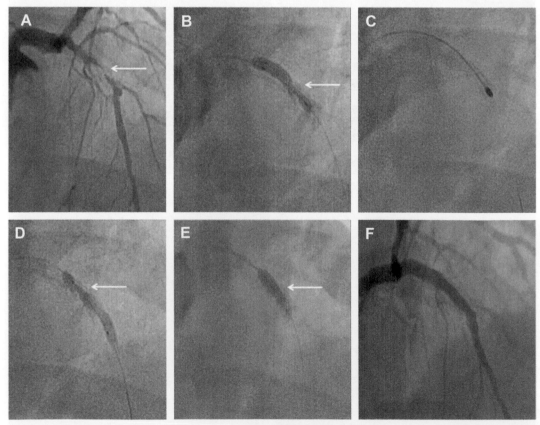

Fig. 8. IVL for unsuccessful rotational atherectomy PCI. (A) Severe proximal LAD stenosis with heavy calcification (arrow). (B) Wasting of a high-pressure noncompliant balloon used for lesion preparation (arrow). (C) Successful rotational atherectomy with a 1.75-mm burr. (D) Evidence of an undilatable lesion despite rotational atherectomy and noncompliant balloon predilatation (arrow). (E) Application of 3.5-mm IVL in the undilated segment with complete balloon dilatation (arrow). (F) Excellent final angiographic result with complete stent expansion after optimization. ([B, C, D, E] Courtesy of Shockwave Medical®, Fremont, CA.)

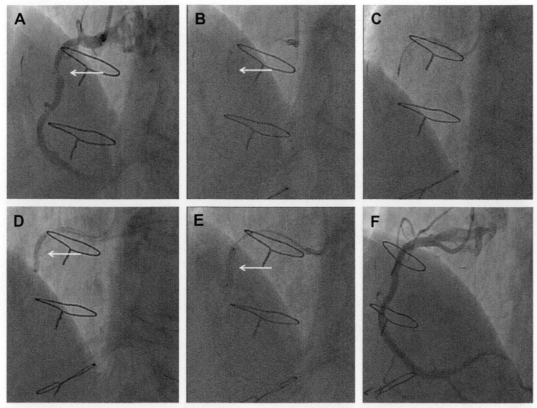

Fig. 9. Rotational atherectomy–facilitated IVL-assisted procedure. (*A*) Severe proximal RCA stenosis in a patient after coronary artery bypass grafting (*arrow*). (*B*) Inability to pass a low-profile balloon despite guide extension catheter support (*arrow*). (*C*) Rotational atherectomy with a 1.5-mm burr. (*D*) Ongoing wasting of the undilatable lesion (*arrow*). (*E*) Application of lithotripsy using a 3.5-mm IVL balloon (*arrow*). (*F*) Excellent angiographic result with complete stent expansion. ([*B, C, D, E*] *Courtesy of* Shockwave Medical®, Fremont, CA.)

calcified lesion, but the catheter could not be delivered to the target lesion. Preparation of the lesion with rotational atherectomy allowed passage of a noncompliant balloon; however, the lesion was still not fully dilatable, and hence IVL was used to allow adequate lesion preparation to avoid stent underexpansion.

Chronic Total Occlusion Percutaneous Coronary Intervention

Advances in PCI for the revascularization of chronic total occlusions (CTOs) have improved the success of connection between the proximal and distal segments of the vessels and subsequent disobliteration. The CTO can be crossed in an antegrade or retrograde fashion by either true-to-true luminal crossing or by first entering the subintimal space, followed by reentry into the true lumen.[24] In the presence of a calcified coronary vessel, connecting these tissue planes can often be problematic, despite attempts to fracture calcification with standard balloon techniques. Given its ability to modify both intimal calcification and deep tissue

calcification, IVL can be a useful tool to modify the calcification and facilitate the proximal and distal vessel connection in order to complete a CTO procedure.[25] **Fig. 10** shows a case in which IVL was used to facilitate revascularization of a right coronary artery CTO using reverse, controlled antegrade retrograde tracking.

Peripheral Use to Aid Large-bore Vascular Access

Use of IVL in the peripheral domain has been well recognized and predates the use of the technology for coronary arterial calcification. Extensive experience exists in the area of peripheral artery intervention with IVL for peripheral vascular disease. This experience includes the Disrupt-PAD (Peripheral Artery Disease) I trial, which is a single-arm, premarket European study that showed the safety and performance of IVL as a standalone therapy in heavily calcified femoral-popliteal lesions at 6-month follow-up.[26] The Disrupt-PAD II trial, a multicenter prospective study of heavily calcified, stenotic,

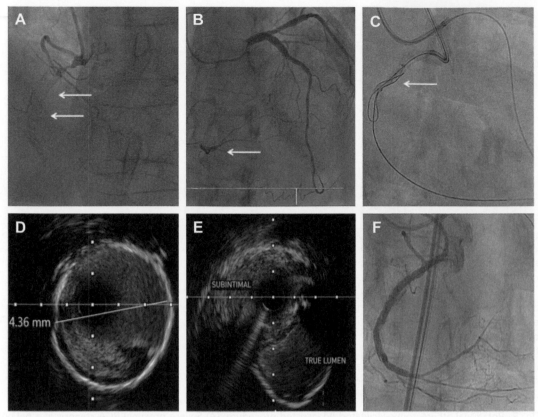

Fig. 10. IVL-assisted CTO PCI procedure. (A) RCA CTO with heavy calcification (arrows). (B) Left-to-right collaterals to the distal RCA (arrow). (C) Application of a 3.0-mm IVL balloon to allow calcium modification and connection between the retrograde and antegrade equipment (arrow). (D) intravascular ultrasonography (IVUS) showing calcification of the proximal RCA. (E) IVUS showing the subintimal space and calcified proximal vessel. (F) Final angiographic result with RCA disobliteration. ([C, D, E] Courtesy of Shockwave Medical®, Fremont, CA; and From Yeoh J, Hill J, Spratt JC. Intravascular lithotripsy assisted chronic total occlusion revascularization with reverse controlled antegrade retrograde tracking. Catheter Cardiovasc Interv 2019; with permission.)

femoropopliteal arteries, showed procedural safety with minimal vessel injury and minimal use of adjunctive stents in a complex, difficult-to-treat population.[27]

Large-bore vascular access for structural intervention can be problematic when extensive atherosclerotic calcification is present in the iliofemoral system and can lead to the need for alternative access sites, such as transaortic, transapical, or transaxillary, or can result in a clinical decision that the patient is not suitable for percutaneous intervention. This situation is often problematic for patients with symptoms and at high surgical risk who may end up being treated medically. IVL of the iliofemoral system has been described as a means to increase the ability to gain successful large-bore vascular access to complete structural intervention.[28] In doing so, IVL may represent a straightforward technique to preserve the benefits of reduced morbidity and mortality of transfemoral transcatheter aortic valve replacement (TAVR) in

patients with calcified peripheral arterial disease.[29] Fig. 11 shows a case in which IVL was used to prepare the iliofemoral system for successful passage of the TAVR sheath.

Iliofemoral calcification can similarly be problematic in patients indicated for high-risk coronary revascularization in the setting of poor ventricular function, because it may preclude placement of large-bore ventricular support catheters. In the setting in which left ventricular support is considered but iliofemoral calcification can prevent insertion of such support, IVL can be useful in increasing the success of large-bore femoral vascular access.[30]

Summary and Discussion for Future Research

To date, clinical data have shown IVL to be a new and novel tool that seems safe and feasible as an adjunct to PCI, particularly for calcified, complex lesions. There is evidence of safety in low-risk patients, but, with increased clinical applicability in

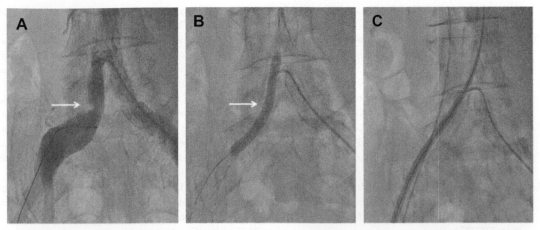

Fig. 11. IVL-assisted large-bore femoral access. (*A*) Iliofemoral angiogram showing a calcified iliac artery with severe stenosis (*arrow*). (*B*) Application of lithotripsy using a 6-mm balloon (*arrow*). (*C*) Passage of the large-bore sheath to facilitate TAVR. (*Courtesy of* Shockwave Medical®, Fremont, CA.)

a broader, all-comers population, accumulated experience will better define real-world procedural and long-term safety. Maturation of the technique and expansion of the technology into mainstream coronary intervention and peripheral intervention for structural procedures will increase as the technology becomes more readily available worldwide.

As the technology of coronary intervention develops, further research will be needed. Such research should focus on the effects of IVL on the polymer characteristics of drug-eluting stents when IVL is used for acute stent underexpansion. Defining the exact benefits of IVL in particular subsets of patients and for defined groups of coronary lesions will be particularly important in left main stem and chronic total occlusion intervention. Direct comparison should be made against the currently available methods of calcium modification in terms of safety, reducing MACEs, and cost-effectiveness. Furthermore, long-term outcomes of IVL in a real-world high-risk population are needed. In addition, and from a global perspective, understanding the role of IVL in coronary calcification will lead to defining appropriate use criteria and incorporation of IVL as part of an algorithm to modify calcium during PCI.

REFERENCES

1. Genereux P, Madhavan MV, Mintz GS, et al. Ischemic outcomes after coronary intervention of calcified vessels in acute coronary syndromes. Pooled analysis from the HORIZONS-AMI (Harmonizing Outcomes With Revascularization and Stents in Acute Myocardial Infarction) and ACUITY (Acute Catheterization and Urgent Intervention Triage Strategy) TRIALS. J Am Coll Cardiol 2014;63: 1845–54.

2. Vandermolen S, Abbott J, De Silva K. What's age got to do with it? A review of contemporary revascularization in the elderly. Curr Cardiol Rev 2015;11: 199–208.

3. Brinton TJ, Ali ZA, Hill JM, et al. Feasibility of shockwave coronary intravascular lithotripsy for the treatment of calcified coronary stenoses. Circulation 2019;139:834–6.

4. Brinton T, Di Mario C, Meredith I, et al. Performance of the lithotripsy system in treating calcified coronary lesions prior to stenting: results from the DISRUPT CAD Study. Transcatheter Cardiovascular Therapeutics paper presented to the Transcatheter Cardiovascular Therapeutics, Washington, DC, October 31, 2016.

5. Ali ZA, Brinton TJ, Hill JM, et al. Optical coherence tomography characterization of coronary lithoplasty for treatment of calcified lesions: first description. JACC Cardiovasc Imaging 2017;10: 897–906.

6. Yeoh J, Pareek N, Arri S. Extending application of intravascular lithotripsy to a high-risk real-world population. JACC Cardiovasc Interv 2019;12:S15.

7. Wong B, El-Jack S, Newcombe R, et al. Shockwave intravascular lithotripsy for calcified coronary lesions: first real-world experience. J Invasive Cardiol 2019;31:46–8.

8. Weisz G, Metzger DC, Liberman HA, et al. A provisional strategy for treating true bifurcation lesions employing a scoring balloon for the side branch: final results of the AGILITY trial. Catheter Cardiovasc Interv 2013;82:352–9.

9. Sakakura K, Inohara T, Kohsaka S, et al. Incidence and determinants of complications in rotational atherectomy: insights from the national clinical

data (J-PCI Registry). Circ Cardiovasc Interv 2016;9 [pii:e004278].

10. Cavusoglu E, Kini AS, Marmur JD, et al. Current status of rotational atherectomy. Catheter Cardiovasc Interv 2004;62:485–98.

11. De Silva K, Roy J, Webb I, et al. A calcific, undilatable stenosis: lithoplasty, a new tool in the box? JACC Cardiovasc Interv 2017;10:304–6.

12. Fujino A, Mintz GS, Matsumura M, et al. A new optical coherence tomography-based calcium scoring system to predict stent underexpansion. EuroIntervention 2018;13:e2182–9.

13. Stone GW, Sabik JF, Serruys PW, et al. Everolimus-eluting stents or bypass surgery for left main coronary artery disease. N Engl J Med 2016;375:2223–35.

14. Makikallio T, Holm NR, Lindsay M, et al. Percutaneous coronary angioplasty versus coronary artery bypass grafting in treatment of unprotected left main stenosis (NOBLE): a prospective, randomised, open-label, non-inferiority trial. Lancet 2016;388: 2743–52.

15. Kang SJ, Ahn JM, Song H, et al. Comprehensive intravascular ultrasound assessment of stent area and its impact on restenosis and adverse cardiac events in 403 patients with unprotected left main disease. Circ Cardiovasc Interv 2011;4:562–9.

16. Kang SJ, Mintz GS, Park DW, et al. Mechanisms of in-stent restenosis after drug-eluting stent implantation: intravascular ultrasound analysis. Circ Cardiovasc Interv 2011;4:9–14.

17. Fitzgerald PJ, Oshima A, Hayase M, et al. Final results of the Can Routine Ultrasound Influence Stent Expansion (CRUISE) study. Circulation 2000;102: 523–30.

18. Kobayashi Y, Okura H, Kume T, et al. Impact of target lesion coronary calcification on stent expansion. Circ J 2014;78:2209–14.

19. Kim JS, Moon JY, Ko YG, et al. Intravascular ultrasound evaluation of optimal drug-eluting stent expansion after poststent balloon dilation using a noncompliant balloon versus a semicompliant balloon (from the Poststent Optimal Stent Expansion Trial [POET]). Am J Cardiol 2008;102:304–10.

20. Kawasaki T, Koga H, Serikawa T, et al. Impact of a prolonged delivery inflation time for optimal drug-eluting stent expansion. Catheter Cardiovasc Interv 2009;73:205–11.

21. Ali ZA, McEntegart M, Hill JM, et al. Intravascular lithotripsy for treatment of stent underexpansion secondary to severe coronary calcification. Eur Heart J 2018. [Epub ahead of print].

22. Salazar C, Escaned J, Tirado G, et al. Undilatable calcific coronary stenosis causing stent underexpansion and late stent thrombosis: a complex scenario successfully managed with intravascular lithotripsy. JACC Cardiovasc Interv 2019. [Epub ahead of print].

23. Tomey MI, Kini AS, Sharma SK. Current status of rotational atherectomy. JACC Cardiovasc Interv 2014;7:345–53.

24. Spratt JC, Strange JW. Retrograde procedural planning, skills development, and how to set up a base of operations. Interv Cardiol Clin 2012;1: 325–38.

25. Yeoh J, Hill J, Spratt JC. Intravascular lithotripsy assisted chronic total occlusion revascularization with reverse controlled antegrade retrograde tracking. Catheter Cardiovasc Interv 2019;93(7): 1295–7.

26. Brinton TJ, Brodmann M, Werner M. Safety and Performance of the Shockwave Medical Lithoplasty® System in treating calcified peripheral vascular lesions: 6-Month Results from the two-phase DISRUPT PAD Study. J Am Coll Cardiol 2016;68:B314.

27. Brodmann M, Werner M, Holden A, et al. Primary outcomes and mechanism of action of intravascular lithotripsy in calcified, femoropopliteal lesions: results of Disrupt PAD II. Catheter Cardiovasc Interv 2019;93:335–42.

28. Di Mario C, Chiriatti N, Stolcova M, et al. Lithotripsy-assisted transfemoral aortic valve implantation. Eur Heart J 2018;39:2655.

29. Di Mario C, Goodwin M, Ristalli F, et al. A prospective registry of intravascular lithotripsy-enabled vascular access for transfemoral transcatheter aortic valve replacement. JACC Cardiovasc Interv 2019;12:502–4.

30. Riley RF, Corl JD, Kereiakes DJ. Intravascular lithotripsy-assisted Impella insertion: a case report. Catheter Cardiovasc Interv 2019;93(7):1317–9.

Printed and bound by CPI Group (UK) Ltd, Croydon, CR0 4YY

03/10/2024

01040307-0006